Table of Contents

Practice Test #1

Practice Questions

1. The OTR asks you to review her evaluation of a patient with Guillain-Barré syndrome. In her evaluation some behaviors she may have observed with the patient are all except one of the following:
    a. The patient was unable to complete the 9-hole peg test because of muscle weakness
    b. The patient reported pain was in her arms and legs
    c. The patient presented with slurred speech
    d. The patient scored low on a Semmes-Weinstein sensory evaluation for her hands

2. The OTR asks you to review her evaluation of a patient with myasthenia gravis. In her evaluation, some behaviors she may have observed with the patient are all except one of the following:
    a. The patient was unable to open and close one eye normally
    b. The patient presented with slurred speech
    c. The patient was unable to chew food for longer than 15 seconds without starting to fatigue
    d. The patient was unable bend down to touch toes because of lack of gross motor control

3. The COTA is treating a patient with ideational apraxia. During the initial treatment session with the COTA, the patient displays one of the following behaviors:
    a. The patient is unable to perform fine motor tasks
    b. The patient is unable to perform gross motor tasks
    c. The patient cannot identify objects with eyes closed
    d. The patient uses a sponge to brush teeth

4. A patient is coming into the facility after being evaluated during the initial visit by the OTR. The COTA has already reviewed the chart and is ready to implement the treatment plan. The OTR has written that the patient is in stage 1 of Brunnstrom's stages of motor recovery. The patient presents with all of the following except:
    a. The patient's biceps reflex is present
    b. The patient's limbs are flaccid and the nervous system is in a state of inhibition
    c. The patient's muscles do not respond to facilitation
    d. The patient's triceps muscle reflex is hypoactive

5. A COTA is treating a patient with a stroke and the patient is at stage 6 on the Brunnstrom's stages of motor recovery. After 6 treatment sessions with the patient, the COTA observes that the patient is now able to complete the treatment activities in the clinic without difficulty and reports to the COTA that he is independent at home with all his activities of daily living/instrumental activities of daily living (ADL/IADL). He has no evidence of functional impairment at this time and activities are at a prestroke level. The COTA's next step should be:
    a. Initiate discharge planning and discharge the patient on the next visit with a home exercise program (HEP)
    b. Call the patient's family to report the gains the patient has made in therapy
    c. Call the physician to report the change of the patient's status
    d. Report to the OTR the patient's new status and change in symptoms and collaborate with the OTR on the next steps in the treatment process for the patient

6. The door swing measurement for a walker is:
   a. 12 inches
   b. 14 inches
   c. 16 inches
   d. 18 inches

7. The door swing measurement for a wheelchair is:
   a. 26 inches
   b. 24 inches
   c. 22 inches
   d. 28 inches

8. What is the ADA requirement for a countertop height?
   a. 29 inches
   b. 30 inches
   c. 31 inches
   d. 32 inches

9. A patient comes in after a stroke. The COTA has read the diagnosis of the stroke is left cerebral vascular accident. The patient has all of the following behaviors except:
   a. The patient is overly cautious of the first treatment activity the COTA has implemented
   b. The patient takes the initiative to start a new treatment activity without prodding
   c. The patient describes how hard it is to complete basic tasks during their day
   d. The patient will not go for a walk alone because of safety fears

10. Which one is a characteristic of the symmetric tonic reflex?
    a. Complete extension of the head, trunk, and extremities
    b. Upright positioning of the head
    c. Arm extension, arm flexion, and adduction
    d. Flexion of hips and knees

11. When is the age of onset of the Landau reflex?
    a. Birth to 2 months
    b. 3 to 4 months
    c. 4 to 6 months
    d. 6 to 8 months

12. A patient comes into the facility wearing a hand-based thumb spica splint. The chart reports no lateral deviation allowed at the metacarpophalangeal (MCP) joint. What might the patient's diagnosis be?
    a. flexor pollicis longus (FPL) repair zone 1
    b. extensor pollicis longus (EPL) repair zone 2
    c. ulnar collateral ligament (UCL) repair
    d. scaphoid fracture

13. An OTR evaluates a patient with a flexor tendon injury who is 2 days postop. The OTR fabricates the splint for the patient and writes a POC in the evaluation process. The patient arrives at the facility the next day to have the treatment plan be implemented by the treating COTA. Upon arrival, the COTA observes the patient not wearing her splint in the waiting room. The COTA's first action should be:

    a. Noting the patient was explained the precautions by the OTR and it is her responsibility to follow the instructions given to her

    b. Call the physician and explain what you saw

    c. Immediately contact the supervising OTR and report that the patient is noncompliant with splint wear and care

    d. Contact the patient's family to see if they can help with overall compliance with wearing the splint

14. A patient is diagnosed with a small rotator cuff repair. The muscle involved in the repair is the supraspinatus muscle. This muscles function is:

    a. external rotation and flexion of the humerus

    b. internal rotation and flexion of the humerus

    c. extension and abduction humerus

    d. flexion and abduction of the humerus

15. There are many ways to gather information on a patient. As a COTA, it is important to be able to gather information in various ways in order to best treat the patient. All of the following are ways to gather data on a patient:

    a. checklists

    b. client/patient records

    c. observation/interview

    d. hearsay from office staff

16. A patient has suffered third-degree burns on over 80% of their right hand. The OTR has already completed the evaluation and fabricated the splint. What position will their right anti-deformity splint be in?

    a. Wrist neutral/ metacarpophalangeal (MP) flexion to 40 degrees of all digits/ thumb flexed to 40 degrees at the MP and slightly adducted

    b .Wrist 30-45 degrees of extension/ MP flexed to 70 degrees all digits/thumb with interphalangeal (IP) extended and abducted

    c .Wrist extended 30-45 degrees of extension/ MPs extended to 0 degrees all digits with thumb out of splint

    d. Wrist neutral/MPs flexed to 70 degrees/thumb MP flexed to 30

17. The COTA has observed a patient complete some basic ADL activities in the clinic. The COTA has determined that the patient has perception deficits. What are some behaviors the COTA might have seen?

    a. Patient is unable to complete any tasks due to both fine and gross motor difficulty

    b. Patient is creating a disorganized space when trying to complete the task, has difficulty scanning the activity needed to complete, and is often acting impulsively

    c. Patient has difficulty with hand-eye coordination during the tasks

    d. Patient has difficulty recognizing objects needed for basic self-care tasks

18. The COTA has been treating a patient post cerebrovascular accident (CVA). The COTA has been working on treatment activities in which the patient's vision is occluded and he must try and identify the object. This COTA is treating a patient with the following problem:
  a. Simultanagnosia
  b. Prosopagnosia
  c. Astereognosis
  d. Graphesthesia

19. A COTA is observing a patient who has an Allen Cognitive Level. The COTA observes the patient understanding tactile cues provided and sees the patient copy the actions of others to complete a task. The patient is able to imitate all three running stitches as related to the assessment. The patient is not able to follow written instructions that are provided for them. What Allen Cognitive Level might this patient be on?
  a. Level 1
  b. Level 6
  c. Level 5
  d. Level 3

20. A COTA is working with a patient to try and gain her independence with brushing her teeth. The COTA has placed the toothpaste and toothbrush next to the sink and asks the patient to complete the task. The patient starts by placing the toothbrush in her mouth without using the toothpaste. What behaviors is this patient exhibiting?
  a. dyspraxia
  b. ideational apraxia
  c. akinesia
  d. dysmetria

21. A patient comes into the clinic with the diagnosis of lateral epicondylitis. The symptoms of the patient's diagnosis are pain along the lateral epicondyle that radiates down to the wrist. The POC is to provide the patient with an elbow strap, ice/deep friction massage, and stretching. How often should this patient be seen in your clinic?
  a. 5 times a week for the first 2 weeks of treatment until patient is pain free
  b. 2 times a week for 6 weeks and then a follow-up with the physician
  c. Let the patient decide how many times he needs to be seen depending on his pain level every day
  d. After the initial visit provide the patient with a good HEP and have him follow up with the physician

22. The COTA is treating a patient with a flexor tendon injury 2 days after surgery. This patient has a zone 2 injury on both his index and middle digits. The flexor digitorum profundus (FDP)/flexor digitorum superficialis (FDS) is affected with a 100% laceration in both fingers. Upon the initial visit it is important to observe all except one of the following in the patient's hand:
  a. edema
  b. check for any signs of infection
  c. active range of motion (AROM) of the digits
  d. passive range of motion (PROM) of the digits

23. Which of the following is not a characteristic of a static splint?
    a. Prevent the patient from moving
    b. Align joints for healing or reducing pain
    c. No moving parts
    d. Moving parts are included

24. Which of the following assessment may be used for a sensory integration (SI) patient?
    a. Kohlman Evaluation of Living Skills (KELS)
    b. Schroeder-Block-Campbell
    c. Jacobs Prevocational Skills Assessment
    d. Allen Cognitive Levels Screen

25. Which one of the following is not in the KELS five areas of living skills?
    a. Safety and health
    b. Work and leisure
    c. Social skills
    d. Transportation and telephone

26. The COTA is preparing to give an assessment to a patient. Which of the following may the COTA do to prepare for the assessment?
    a. Prepare the environment for the assessment, have the patient complete the assessment, score and interpret the results of the assessment.
    b. Communicate to the patient the intent of the assessment and explain instructions, collaborate with the OTR on scoring and interpretation of results, and review the POC with the patient.
    c. Contact the physician regarding the date and time of when the assessment will be given, schedule the assessment with another patient with the same diagnosis, and interpret the results with the OTR
    d. Review and collect evaluation data to decide if an assessment is appropriate without the input from to OTR, prepare the environment for the assessment, and interpret the results

27. Which one of the following is not an example of interview style assessments?
    a. Rating Scale Activity Configuration
    b. Prevocational Inventory
    c. Allen Cognitive Screen
    d. Sensorimotor History

28. A COTA's role in giving assessments involves all except one of the following:
    a. Collects data as instructed by the OTR
    b. Organizes information gathered and reports it to the OTR
    c. Scores and interprets results
    d. Establishes service competency

29. The COTA is observing a patient in the clinic with a spinal cord injury. The patient is able to complete tasks that involve elbow extension, active finger extension using the tenodesis grasp, and wrist flexion. What level of spinal cord injury (SCI) does this patient have?
    a. C7
    b. C6
    c. C5
    d. C4

30. The COTA is observing a patient in the clinic with a spinal cord injury. The patient is seen using a dorsal wrist splint with universal cuff, Dycem to stabilize his plate, and a long straw with a straw holder. What level SC may this patient be?
  a. C7
  b. C5
  c. C1
  d. C8/T1

31. A patient comes in with a radial nerve injury. He has lost function of his ECRL/ECRB and EDC muscles. He is unable to move his wrist and digits. He is currently wearing a wrist and finger extension splint for increased function until these muscles regenerate. What muscle grade may he have?
  a. Grade 3
  b. Grade 4
  c. Grade 2
  d. Grade 0

32. The COTA is reviewing the evaluation administered by the OTR before beginning treatment on a patient with a diagnosis of flexor carpi radialis (FCR) tendonitis. The chart reports the manual muscle testing (MMT) of the FCR to be 2+. What might the patient's ROM status be?
  a. Patient is able to move through full ROM both with and against gravity
  b. Patient can move through incomplete ROM with gravity eliminated
  c. Patient can move through incomplete ROM (more than 50%) against gravity
  d. Patient is able to move through incomplete ROM (less than 50%) against gravity or through complete ROM in gravity-eliminated plane with slight resistance

33. The same patient with the FCR tendonitis diagnosis has now been treated in the clinic for 4 weeks. His muscle grade has now increased to Fair Plus. The patient can now partially move through complete ROM against gravity with slight resistance. What MMT grade would you record in the chart?
  a. Grade 3
  b. Grade 3+
  c. Grade 4
  d. Grade 4+

34. A patient comes in with a diagnosis of traumatic brain injury (TBI) and a Rancho Level 4. What behaviors might this patient have?
  a. Confused, inappropriate, nonagitated/needs max assist/appears alert
  b. Confused, agitated/needs max assist/disorientated/short attention span/inappropriate behavior
  c. No response total assist needed/unresponsive to all stimuli
  d. Localized response total assist/responds to some commands/may respond to discomfort

35. What are the adult standard wheelchair dimensions?
  a. Width 20"/depth 16"/height 22"
  b. Width 18"/depth 16"/height 20"
  c. Width 20"/depth 19"/height 22"
  d. Width 18"/depth 18"/height 22"

36. What are the ramp slope measurements?
    a. 1" vertical rise to 12"
    b. 2" vertical rise to 12"
    c. 1" vertical rise to 14"
    d. 1" vertical rise to 16"

37. A patient enters the rehab facility with a diagnosis of a total hip replacement (THR) 1 week postop. All of the following are precautions of this diagnosis except for:
    a. No hip flexion greater then 90
    b. No internal rotation
    c. No external rotation
    d. No extension

38. Which one of the following statements is an untrue description of an IEP?
    a. Individualized Education Plan
    b. Geared to treat 3 to 18 year olds with a focus on education
    c. Performed in a hospital setting
    d. Performed in a school setting

39. When writing notes to document a patient's treatment, which of the following would not fit into the O portion of the note?
    a. How much assistance the patient needed to complete the task
    b. What the patient completed in treatment that day
    c. The clinician's view of how the treatment session went
    d. The exact parameters for the modality used in treatment

40. The COTA is treating a child to work on her pre-writing skills. The child holds the pencil with a fisted hand in a power-like grasp. The pencil is located on the ulnar side of the hand and writes on the paper as the arm and hand move around in a unit. The child is 1½ years old. The grasp the child is using is:
    a. Palmer-supinated grasp
    b. Digital-pronated grasp
    c. Static tripod posture grasp
    d. Dynamic tripod posture grasp

41. A patient enters the clinic with complaints of pain and numbness on the ulnar side of their hand. He reports that the pain and numbness increase at night when he is sleeping. The physician diagnosed cubital tunnel. What splint would this patient need?
    a. Wrist cock-up
    b. Dynamic wrist/finger extension splint
    c. Pinky/Ring finger flexion splint
    d. Elbow splint to prevent extreme positions of elbow flexion

42. A patient presents with hyperextension of their fourth and fifth digits metacarpophalangeal joints or "claw hand deformity." This is a characteristic of which diagnosis:
    a. Boutonniere deformity
    b. Swan neck deformity
    c. Ulnar nerve injury
    d. Median nerve injury

43. A COTA is treating a patient with a diagnosis of graphesthesia. Which one of the following behaviors would not be observed?
   a. Inability to identify forms
   b. Inability to identify body parts
   c. Inability to identify numbers
   d. Inability to identify letters

44. Which one of the following describes Central Cord Syndrome?
   a. Often results from hyperextension injuries and a patient will have more upper extremity (UE) injuries than lower extremity (LE).
   b. Often results from ipsilateral spastic paralysis in which a patient loses a position of sense, has contralateral loss of pain, and loss of thermal sense.
   c. Often results from flexion injuries in which a patient loses bilateral motor function. Patients lose pain, temperature, and touch sensation.
   d. Often result from injury of the sacral cord and lumbar nerve roots. Patients have LE motor and sensory loss.

45. The COTA is treating a patient who has a diagnosis spinal cord injury (SCI) level C1-C3. The behaviors the patient has are:
   a. Patient has a limited movement of head and neck and is on a ventilator to breathe. Talking for this patient can be difficult and limited and patients often need a mouth stick.
   b. Patient has head and neck control and the ability to shrug shoulders
   c. Patient can shrug shoulders, bend elbows, and supinate and pronate forearm
   d. Patient has normal motor function in the head, neck, shoulders, and arms

46. The supervising OTR has gone on vacation for a few days. The COTA is going to perform treatment for established patients who have already been evaluated by the OTR and have an established treatment plan in place. While the OTR is out, a new patient arrives at the facility and needs an evaluation performed to determine if OT services are needed. What should the COTA do?
   a. Evaluate the patient to determine if OT services are needed. The COTA has worked at the facility for a few years and is knowledgeable of the evaluation process.
   b. Reschedule the evaluation for when the OTR arrives back from vacation
   c. Call the referring physician to check if it is okay for the COTA to perform the evaluation
   d. Inform the patient's family that you have been working at the facility for many years and are comfortable performing the evaluation to determine if OT services are needed.

47. A TBI patient is ready for discharge as determined by the OTR. The patient is going home to live with his sister, brother-in-law, and their three small children. The patient has been given an HEP for home follow-through with his therapy program and will be returning to the facility on an outpatient basis. The patient and his sister's family are coming to the last therapy visit to review the HEP for home and how the family can safely prepare their home. The COTA's emphasis on this visit should be:
   a. Communicate to the patient and the patient's family the discharge plans, review the HEP provided, and instruct them on how to modify their home for a safe transition home.
   b. Reschedule a re-evaluation with the patient's family for a week after the patient has been home
   c. Provide the patient's family with the physician's number in case there is a problem with the transition
   d. Instruct the patient's family that TBI patients should not be left alone with small children

48. A patient is admitted to a skilled nursing facility (SNF) with congestive heart failure (CHF) level 4. What symptoms will he display?
 a. Slightly limited in performing ADLs/IADLs
 b. No limitation in ADLs/IADLs by pain, palpitations, or angina
 c. Limited while performing physical activities and also during less strenuous activities while experiencing symptoms
 d. Unable to perform any physical activities without experiencing symptoms and often has symptoms at rest

49. A patient is being evaluated by the OTR. She is reporting pain and numbness in her thumb, index, and middle fingers. She said these symptoms are often worse at night and when she is using the computer for long periods of time. Which diagnosis best describes what this patient has:
 a. Radial tunnel syndrome
 b. Cubital tunnel syndrome
 c. Carpal tunnel syndrome
 d. De Quervain syndrome

50. A patient comes into the clinic with a diagnosis of a TBI. The COTA observes that she is not able to identify her own body parts or other patient's body parts in the clinic. This is called:
 a. Prosopagnosia
 b. Simultanagnosia
 b. Graphesthesia
 c. Autotopagnosia

51. The COTA is reading a patient's chart before initiating treatment activities for the patient to perform. In the chart it states that the patient's ROM is WFL. What does WFL mean?
 a. Within function limits
 b. Within function level
 c. Within fracture limitations
 d. Without fracture limitations

52. A SOAP note stands for:
 a. Supportive, Objective, Assessment, and Plan
 b. Subjective, Objective, Assessment, and Plan
 c. Subjective, Observable, Assessment, and Plan
 d. Subjective, Observable, Accurate, and Plan

53. A COTA just started working at a SNF. The COTA is performing chart reviews on patients that he is going to treat in the upcoming week. All of the following should be indicated in the patient's health record except for:
 a. What happened and what was reported
 b. What services were provided and where/when these services were provided
 c. An assessment of how the client responded to the services provided
 d. A full report from the patient's employer on job duties he used to perform

54. All of the following are side effects of tricyclic antidepressants except for:
 a. Postural hypotension
 b. Muscle twitching
 c. Seizures
 d. Urinary retention

55. Which of the following symptoms are the side effects of monoamine oxidase inhibitors (MAOIs)?
    a. Constipation, seizures, slurred speech
    b. Sweating, palpations, increase in BP
    c. Urinary retention, constipation, sexual dysfunction
    d. Shivering, tremors, anxiety

56. A COTA is working in an inpatient mental health facility. She has been treating a patient with fugue syndrome. What behaviors might this patient exhibit?
    a. Restricted emotion
    b. Decreased speech and cognitive ability
    c. Inability to socialize in a group setting
    d. Take on a new identity of a family member

57. A patient presents with a middle finger deformity. This is causing the patient's finger to hyperextend at the proximal interphalangeal (PIP) and flex at the distal interphalangeal (DIP). This deformity is called:
    a. Boutonniere deformity
    b. Swan neck deformity
    c. Osteoarthritis deformity
    d. Rheumatoid deformity

58. A COTA is asked by the supervising OTR to perform a COPM (Canadian Occupational Performance Measure) on a patient who has been diagnosed with a TBI and is going to be discharged to an outpatient facility. What areas will the COTA measure during this assessment?
    a. Self-care, productivity, and leisure skills
    b. Self-care, vocational tasks, and leisure skills
    c. Social, leisure, and functional ROM abilities
    d. Vocational, safety knowledge, and leisure activities

59. A COTA has recently accepted a position at an outpatient hand facility working under an OTR/CHT. The COTA is observing the OTR treat patients the first few days before she is allowed to start treating her first patient. She observes the OTR treating patients who present with decreased ROM, strength, and endurance, preventing full function for the individual. What FOR is the OTR using to treat these patients?
    a. Motor Skills Acquisition
    b. Biomechanical
    c. Psychodynamic
    d. Role Acquisition

60. Which of the following is not an example of a performance skill?
    a. Motor and praxis skills
    b. Social skills
    c. Vocational performance
    d. Cognitive skills

61. A COTA is treating a patient with a TBI whose level of cognition has decreased significantly over the past week; the COTA is concerned about the safety of the patient. What should the COTA's next step be?
    a. Call the patient's family to discuss the changes observed
    b. Call the social worker involved in the case to address the safety concerns
    c. Report immediately to the supervising OTR to address the safety issues
    d. Talk to the patient to discuss your concerns and to see if the patient can understand the safety concerns you have

62. A COTA is allowed to fill all of the following roles except for:
    a. Practitioner
    b. Teacher
    c. Peer Educator
    d. Evaluator

63. What would be an appropriate goal for a patient with a C5 SCI?
    a. Max A for both UE and LE
    b. Mod A with UE/Max A with LE
    c. Min A with UE/Mod A with LE
    d. Mod A with UE/Mod A with LE

64. Which of the following would be an appropriate goal for a patient with a SCI C1-C3?
    a. Will be able to direct others for all applicable care including pressure relief, UE ROM techniques, and UE positioning in bed and wheelchair
    b. Independent with wheelchair propulsion inside on hard level surfaces
    c. Independent with power recline/tilt wheelchair
    d. Minimal assistance with self-care activities

65. A COTA is treating a pediatric patient who is using the palmer grasp. This patient is holding toys in her palm with fingers on top of the toy and thumb adducted. What age is this grasp typically present?
    a. 4 months
    b. 5 months
    c. 8 months
    d. 6 months

66. A COTA is working in an outpatient hand clinic. Typically patients are seen at this clinic 2 times/week or 3 times/week. When may a patient be seen 5 times/week?
    a. If the patient reports they are having a lot of pain and requests to be seen 5 times/week
    b. If the patient is postop and nervous about going a few days between appointments
    c. If the patient presents with an open infection and the wound needs to be evaluated and redressed every 24 hours
    d. If the patient reports he is going to be noncompliant with their HEP

67. The COTA is reading the referral from the physician regarding a patient with a flexor tendon repair. The physician states he wants to use the Kleinert protocol for flexor tendon repair. Which ROM exercise would be appropriate to have the patient perform at 0-4 weeks postop?
    a. Passive flexion of all digits into palm
    b. Passive flexion and active extension exercises within the confines of the splint
    c. Active flexion and extension exercises
    d. Passive flexion and passive extension exercises within the confines of the splint

68. A COTA is treating a patient for oculomotor deficits. What treatment activities would be appropriate for this patient?
    a. Fine motor (FM)/gross motor (GM) activities, LE adaptive equipment training, and cognitive perceptual activities
    b. Eye movement activities, scanning tasks, visio-motor tasks, and activities to increase endurance during tasks
    c. Providing patient with community resources, larger prints when reading, and magnification
    d. Activities that decrease patterns, adapt environment for safety, and change color to increase contrast

69. The COTA is trying to come up with activities for a patient with astereognosis. What activities would be best for a patient with this diagnosis?
    a. Vision occluded, the patient must identify objects in a bucket of rice
    b. Vision occluded, the patient must write down characteristics of self
    c. Vision occluded, the patient must perform FM/GM tasks
    d. Vision allowed, the patient must identify objects presented

70. An OTR is treating a patient with a C4 SCI. The OTR asked you to provide the patient with some adaptive equipment to help increase his function. What equipment may you choose?
    a. Dorsal wrist splint with universal cuff
    b. A ratchet splint
    c. Long straw with a straw holder
    d. Suspension sling

71. A patient with decreased sensation comes into the clinic following a peripheral nerve injury to his right hand. The patient cannot distinguish between hot/ cold or deep pressure/light touch. What are some appropriate treatment activities for this patient?
    a. Use of modalities such as ultrasound/hot packs
    b. Electrical stimulation to the extensor/flexor muscle groups
    c. Sensory buckets such a rice and popcorn
    d. Resting hand splint for anti-deformity positioning

72. A patient comes into the clinic with a hypersensitive scar following an open carpal tunnel release. What treatment activities may be appropriate for this patient?
    a. Iontophoresis using dexamethasone
    b. Ultrasound as a thermal modality
    c. Sensory buckets such as cotton balls and pasta
    d. Wrist brace to protect scar

73. A COTA is treating a patient with a metabolic equivalent (MET) level of 1.4-2. What treatment activities would be appropriate for this patient?
    a. Have the patient stand while showering and bathing independently
    b. Have the patient perform balance exercises on a mat and begin ambulation exercises
    c. Have the patient sit while performing light ADLs
    d. Have the patient stand while washing dishes and making beds

74. Which of the following POC makes the most sense when treating a patient with a diagnosis of Dupuytren disease postoperatively?
    a. PROM exercises and flexion splint with the MPs at 70 degrees
    b. Extension splint for all digits wearing it at all times for 2 weeks
    c. No splinting, just begin gentle AROM exercises to all digits
    d. No splinting, just scar management technique and gentle AROM as tolerated

75. A COTA is treating a pediatric patient 6 to 7 months old. The COTA is working on his fine motor skills and self-feeding goals. What treatment activities would be appropriate for this patient?
    a. Have the child drink from a cup independently
    b. Use a spoon and bring food to mouth
    c. Bang the spoon on the table
    d. Pick up Cheerios from table and place in mouth

76. Which of the following treatment activities would be appropriate for a 4-month-old infant who is working on achieving developmental milestones?
    a. Picking up objects placed on floor when the child is seated
    b. Place object at the child's midline and have her reach for it as she is supine
    c. Place the child prone and have her pick up small toys using the radial palmer grasp
    d. Have the child work on pincer grasp while supine

77. Which of the following is not a proper adaptive equipment option for a patient with a C6 SCI?
    a. Ucuff
    b. Cup with long handle
    c. Rocker knife
    d. Long-handled straw

78. The COTA is treating a patient who is in a wheelchair. After the treatment session the COTA has transferred the patient back to his wheelchair and noticed the patient is leaning forward too far in the seat. What does this indicate?
    a. Armrests are too high
    b. Armrests are too low
    c. Footrests need to be lowered
    d. Footrests need to be higher

79. Which of the following would be appropriate treatment activities for a patient with a FCR MMT grade of 3+?
    a. In a gravity-eliminated plane, have patient reach for cones
    b. Have the patient pick up cones against gravity
    c. Have the patient do 3lb wrist curls against gravity
    d. Neuromuscular electrical stimulation (NMES) to FCR to facilitate ROM in a gravity-eliminated plane

80. A COTA is evaluating the home of a patient who is about to be discharged from an inpatient facility to his own home. He uses a wheelchair and needs his home to be modified to allow him to get around safely. The doorway does not allow for his wheelchair to go through because it is only 31½ inches wide. What may the COTA do to modify the door so that the wheelchair can safely pass through?

    a. Remove the doorstops

    b. Create a door divider where the top and bottom open separately

    c. Change the door handles

    d. Remove the outside moldings

81. The COTA is trying to grade an activity to make it harder for a patient who is suffering from a TBI. This patient is working on self-care activities such as brushing hair and brushing teeth in the clinic. The patient has achieved the goal of being able to complete self-care activities independently if all objects are placed on the counter in the correct sequence they are to be used in. What would be the most appropriate way to grade this activity to make it more challenging for the patient?

    a. Give the patient one verbal clue when trying to complete the task

    b. Provide the patient with written instructions she must follow to complete the task

    c. Hide all objects needed to complete task for the patient to find them and complete the activity

    d. Reorganize the objects so that they are not in the correct sequence on the counter and see if the patient can complete the task

82. The COTA is treating a cardiac rehab patient with a 5-6 MET level. What activities are most appropriate for a patient with this level?

    a. Walking 3.5 mph, cycling 8 mph, golf, and dancing

    b. Digging in a garden, walking 4 mph, cycling 10 mph, and canoeing 4 mph

    c. Shoveling 10 min (22lb), walking 5 mph, cycling 11 mph, and light downhill skiing

    d. Carrying 175 lb, sawing hardwood, jogging 5 mph

83. A COTA is working in an inpatient facility treating SCI patients. The COTA is up on the patient's floor treating the patient in his room. The patient begins to exhibit behaviors associated with autonomic dysreflexia. What should the COTA's next step be?

    a. Leave the patient and immediately report to the supervising OTR what behaviors you have observed

    b. Try to lay the patient down until the symptoms subside

    c. Have the patient immediately place bilateral hands overhead

    d. Immediately use the phone call box in the room to call for medical assistance

84. The COTA is treating a patient with a SCI. All of the following are precautions and contraindications associated with this diagnosis except for:

    a. Osteoporosis

    b. Rheumatoid arthritis (RA)

    c. Pressure ulcers

    d. Thermal dysregulation

85. A COTA is treating a patient with central cord syndrome. What would be the most appropriate treatment activities for this patient?

    a. Bike for 5 min/walk on treadmill at 2 mph

    b. UE arm bike for 5 min/9- hole peg test/cone activity

    c. Bike for 10 min/GM activities for the LE

    d. Adaptive equipment training using a long-handled shoe horn and sock aid

86. A COTA has a patient with decreased both FM and GM skills needed to perform dressing tasks. Which one of the following is not an adaptation to increase function with dressing tasks:
    a. Oversized shirts and dresses
    b. Pants and skirts with elastic waistbands
    c. Long-handled shoe horn
    d. C-bar splint

87. A COTA is treating a patient diagnosed with Parkinson disease. This patient has some balance and coordination issues that are making it difficult for her to perform ADL tasks. Which treatment activities would be most appropriate for this patient?
    a. ROM of UE/LE, strengthening exercises, energy conservation techniques, and safety modifications to patient's environment
    b. Cognitive-skill training, anger management groups, and time management groups
    c. Visual-perceptual activities, FM activities, and anger management groups
    d. Sensory integration techniques, visual-motor activities, cognitive perceptual activities

88. During a child's first year of life it is important to work on functional movement skills such as rolling, head control, learning to sit, and cruising. Which other developmental milestone is important during birth to 12 months of age?
    a. Learning the alphabet
    b. Learning numbers to 10
    c. Crawling
    d. Finger painting

89. A COTA is working on pre-writing skills with a child 2 to 3 years old. All of the following are appropriate activities for this age group except for:
    a. Using broken crayons, have the child hold crayon with thumb and fingers instead of fist
    b. Roll, squeeze, and pull putty
    c. Trace over letters in the alphabet
    d. Finger painting

90. A COTA is treating a child who is tactile defensive. What is the best way to approach this child in a room?
    a. From behind and apply light touch to his shoulder
    b. From behind and apply a firm touch to his shoulder
    c. From the front and apply a firm touch to his shoulder
    d. From the front and apply a light touch to his shoulder

91. Which of the following is not an appropriate treatment activity for a patient who is tactile defensive?
    a. A weighted vest or garment
    b. Use a brush to brush his/her arms and legs
    c. Finger painting
    d. 9-hole peg test for FM dexterity

92. The COTA is treating a child who has a sensitivity to sound and is easily distracted by auditory stimulation. All of the following are appropriate treatment activities/environmental modifications except for:

a. Earplugs for school

b. In the classroom, place child away from the auditory source

c. Prepare child for noisy situations ahead of time

d. In the classroom, place the child near the auditory source so he can get used to the sound

93. A COTA is treating a child who is hypersensitive orally or "orally defensive." Which of the following treatment activities is not appropriate for this child?

a. Finger paint with different foods like pudding, whipped cream, or applesauce

b. Stoke the child before eating a meal with firm pressure around the mouth and face

c. Blow through a straw to race ping pong balls or cotton balls

d. Take food the child does not like and place it in her mouth to get her used to the texture

94. The COTA is treating a small 5-year-old child who is overly sensitive to certain sensory stimuli within their environment. The child is unable to focus in a classroom environment and often appears agitated, restless, and controlling. All of the following are examples of appropriate treatment techniques except for:

a. Gentle slow rocking in a hammock or rocking chair

b. Anger management groups to develop coping skills

c. Squeeze Theraputty or foam ball

d. Wrap up snuggly in a beach towel or blanket

95. The OTR is treating a child who presents with decreased fine motor strength. This child is 7 years old and is having difficulty writing for long periods of time in school. All of the following are appropriate treatment activities to increase FM strength except for which one:

a. Spray bottles/squirt guns

b. Hide objects in Theraputty and have the child try and pull them out

c. Place clothespins around an index card

d. Provide an adaptive pencil holder

96. A COTA is trying to modify a patient's workspace so that it will decrease pressure on his body and adhere to ergonomic guidelines. What is the best position for the patient's knees, hips, and elbows?

a. Flexion 90 degrees hips/80 degrees knees/45 degrees elbows

b. Flexion 80 degrees hips/80 degrees knees/80 degrees elbows

c. Flexion 90 degrees hips/90 degrees knees/90 degrees elbows

d. Flexion 100 degrees hips/100 degrees knees/100 degrees elbows

97. A COTA is treating a patient with a diagnosis of distal radius fracture open reduction and internal fixation (ORIF). This patient is 6 weeks postop and the COTA is about to perform an ultrasound treatment. What would be the most appropriate precaution for this patient during ultrasound?

a. Avoid metal implant

b. Avoid entire dorsal surface of wrist

c. Avoid entire volar surface of wrist

d. Avoid supinator muscle

98. A COTA is treating a patient with muscular dystrophy. All of the following are appropriate treatment activities except for:
    a. FM tasks
    b. GM tasks
    c. Nerve blocks
    d. Adaptive techniques

99. A COTA is trying to write some short-term goals for a patient. The COTA is going to write these goals based on client factors. Which one of the following is not a client factor?
    a. Abilities of the patient
    b. Characteristics of the patient
    c. Beliefs of the patient
    d. Beliefs of the patient's family

100. A patient enters a facility with a diagnosis of complex regional pain syndrome (CRPS). The patient is reporting burning pain in the extremity and the COTA has observed some muscle atrophy. The affected arm feels hot to touch and the skin appears red and blotchy. What would some appropriate treatment activities be for this patient?
    a. Aggressive ROM and strength training
    b. Sensory intergradation techniques and aggressive PROM
    c. Adaptive techniques, patient education, and gentle ROM as tolerated
    d. Strengthening exercises and balance/coordination activities

101. A ulnar nerve laceration can affect the patient's upper extremities differently depending on the exact location of the laceration. Which one of the following would not be an appropriate splint for an ulnar nerve injury?
    a. Dorsal wrist splint with wrist positioned in 30 degrees of flexion
    b. Elbow splint at 90 degrees of flexion combined with wrist flexion splint
    c. MCP flexion block splint
    d. Dynamic extension splint

102. A median nerve laceration can affect the patient's upper extremities differently depending on where the nerve is lacerated. Which one of the following would not be an appropriate splint for a median nerve injury?
    a. Dorsal wrist splint in neutral
    b. Dorsal wrist splint with wrist positioned in 30 degrees of flexion
    c. Elbow splint at 90 degrees of flexion with wrist splint 30 degrees of flexion
    d. C-bar splint

103. A physician has authorized the need for you to fabricate a serial splint to increase ROM in a patient's PIP flexion contracture of their middle finger. How would you explain to the patient what this protocol involves?
    a. Wearing a splint with moveable parts for a short amount of time during the day
    b. Wearing a splint for long periods of time that maintains the same position of the joint.
    c. Wearing a splint for a long period of time while providing a small amount of tension to the joint and adjusting the splint as tolerated to increase the patient's mobility.
    d. Wearing a splint a short period of time and adjusting the splint as tolerated to increase the patient's mobility.

104. All of the following are the purposes of a wrist cock-up splint except:
    a. Allows full MCP flexion while keeping the functional position of the hand and wrist
    b. Positions wrist to decrease pressure on the carpel tunnel
    c. Provides rest and relief of symptoms to the wrist in acute rheumatoid arthritis
    d. Aids with claw deformity of the hand

105. The OTR is treating a patient using the Rood facilitation techniques. The patient has hypertonicity. What treatment technique would best help this patient?
    a. Slow rolling/rocking
    b. Fast rocking
    c. Neck co-contraction
    d. Noxious stimulation

106. The COTA is using Rood facilitation techniques to treat a patient who presents with flaccidly post-CVA. All of the following are examples of facilitatory techniques to help this patient except for:
    a. Tapping
    b. Noxious odor
    c. Painful stimuli
    d. Slow stroking

107. The COTA is using Rood facilitation techniques when treating a patient post-CVA who is spastic. All of the following are examples of inhibitory techniques to help treat this patient except for:
    a. Heavy joint compression
    b. Pleasant odors/perfume
    c. Slow rocking
    d. Slow rolling

108. A COTA is treating a patient who is diagnosed with severe dementia. All of the following are behaviors and risks associated with this disease except for:
    a. Falls
    b. Uncooperative
    c. Wandering
    d. Seizures

109. When an assessment needs to be given to a patient, all of the following are the roles of the COTA except for:
    a. Organizes the information and reports it to the OTR
    b. Documents the assessment
    c. Organizes, analyzes, and interprets the assessment independent of the OTR
    d. Collects information from observation, interviews, and charts

110. The COTA is reviewing a chart on a patient in a coma. This patient has a 4 with best verbal response on the Glasgow Coma Scale. What behaviors might the patient exhibit?
    a. No response with verbal behavior
    b. Incomprehensible sound
    c. Oriented to time, date, and place
    d. Confused but verbal

111. A COTA is treating a patient in a coma and is observing his eye response behaviors. This patient is able to open his eyes in response to painful stimuli. What number on the Glasgow Coma Scale would this patient receive?
    a. 1
    b. 2
    c. 3
    d. 4

112. A COTA is treating a patient with akathisia. What would be the best environment for the patient to maximize performance during treatment?
    a. Use the treatment room when it has a lot of patients in it
    b. Cafeteria during lunchtime
    c. Calm and relaxing environment without a lot of distraction
    d. Group treatments with a lot of people

113. A COTA is treating a patient who is not being cooperative during the treatment tasks. The patient is continuously mimicking the COTA's movements and behaviors instead of completing the task. What type of behavior is this patient exhibiting?
    a. Ideational apraxia
    b. Echopraxia
    c. Prosopagnosia
    d. Anosognosia

114. The COTA is working on color agnosia with a patient. Which one of the following is not an appropriate treatment technique?
    a. Have the patient organize different color blocks together by color
    b. Have the patient use crayons to color a picture that labels what color needs to be used for each part
    c. Holding up different colored flashcards and having the patient name the color they see
    d. Have the patient organize different blocks together by color and verbalize what color each group is

115. The COTA is treating a patient with an Allen Cognitive Level of 3. Which one of the following would not be an appropriate treatment activity?
    a. Demonstrate a simple cooking task and have the patient then perform the same task
    b. Write down the steps to complete a simple self-care task
    c. Ask the patient to show you how to don/doff his shirt
    d. Show the patient how to brush his teeth and have him then repeat the same task

116. A COTA is working with a group of patients with the goal of therapy to increase the awareness of thoughts, needs, feelings, and values through the process of choosing, planning, and implementing an activity. The COTA is working on what type of group:
    a. Task-oriented group
    b. Topical group
    c. Instrumental group
    d. Thematic group

117. A COTA is running a group in which members are discussing what needs to be done in order to complete a cooking task. Each member is helping determine the needed steps in order to make a deli sandwich. The COTA is having each member say one step in the correct sequence necessary to complete the task. This is an example of which type of group:
   a. Task-oriented group
   b. Topical group
   c. Instrumental group
   d. Thematic group

118. A patient needs a resting hand splint. All of the following are appropriate characteristics of this splint except for:
   a. Static splint for wrist, hand, and thumb
   b. Used to immobilize the wrist, hand, and thumb
   c. Used to position the fingers in a lengthened position to prevent deformity
   d. Used to increase mobility of the wrist and hand

119. A patient comes into the clinic with a diagnosis of De Quervain disease. Which splint would be most appropriate for this patient?
   a. Wrist cock-up
   b. C-bar splint
   c. Thumb spica with wrist in 15 degrees of flexion
   d. Thumb spica with wrist in 15 degrees of extension

120. A COTA is treating a child who is 3½ years old. The COTA is working to get the child to use scissors appropriately for the child's age level. All of the following are good treatment activities except for:
   a. Have the child cut the paper in a straight line
   b. Have the child cut simple geometric shapes
   c. Have the child open and close the scissors correctly without paper
   d. Have the child cut complex figure shapes

121. A COTA is treating a patient with a MET level of 1.4 -2. All of the following are appropriate treatment activities except for:
   a. Have the patient sit and brush teeth
   b. Have the patient walk across the room at a slow pace
   c. Gentle isometrics to the patient's UE
   d. Have the patient complete a craft activity while sitting

122. A COTA is working with a 5-month-old infant. The COTA is trying to figure out if the appropriate reflexes are present in the child. The COTA places the infant in a crawling position and extends the head of the child. The child's hips and knees flex. This is an example of which reflex:
   a. Landau reflex
   b. Symmetric tonic reflex
   c. Labyrinthine righting reflex
   d. Moro reflex

123. A patient came in with a diagnosis of skier's thumb. Which splint would be most appropriate for this patient?
    a. Wrist cock-up
    b. MP block for ring/pinky fingers
    c. Hand-based thumb spica
    d. Forearm-based thumb spica

124. The COTA is working with a 3-month-old infant. The COTA is holding the infant vertically and tilting the child's body slowly backwards, forwards, and side to side. Which reflex is the COTA working on?
    a. Landau reflex
    b. Labyrinthine righting reflex
    c. Moro reflex
    d. Galant reflex

125. A patient comes to the clinic with a diagnosis of a medium rotator cuff tear of the supraspinatus muscle. This patient had surgery to repair rotator cuff and is 7 days postop. This patient is currently wearing a sling at all times. What would an appropriate treatment activity be?
    a. AROM all shoulder planes: flexion/extension/internal rotation (IR)/external rotation (ER)/abduction
    b. PROM all shoulder planes: flexion/extension/IR/ER/abduction
    c. No ROM to shoulder joint just unaffected joints
    d. Active-assisted range of motion (AAROM) to all shoulder planes: flexion/extension/IR/ER

126. A COTA is treating a patient with contrast sensitivity deficits. What would be some appropriate treatment techniques?
    a. Change color to increase contrast, decrease patterns, and reduce clutter
    b. Blend color to decrease contrast, increase patterns, and increase clutter
    c. Eye movement activities, visual-motor tasks, and scanning tasks
    d. Scanning training, safety adaptations, and increase lighting in room

127. A COTA is working with a patient who has oculomotor deficits. What would some appropriate treatment techniques be?
    a. Visual-motor tasks, eye movement activities, and scanning tasks
    b. Provide large print, yellow and amber sunglasses, and increase lighting in room
    c. Magnification, larger print, and community resources
    d. Change color to increase contrast, decrease patterns, and reduce clutter

128. A COTA is treating a patient with an MMT of the ECRL/ECRB of 2-. What would be the most appropriate treatment activity to work on these muscles?
    a. Against gravity stack 10 cones together
    b. In a gravity-eliminated plane pick up soup cans
    c. In a gravity-eliminated plane extend wrist backwards 10 times
    d. Against gravity extend wrist backwards 10 times

129. A patient comes into the clinic with a MMT of the FCR of 0. Which one of the following would be an appropriate treatment activity?
    a. In a gravity-eliminated plane have the patient flex the wrist 5 times
    b. Against gravity have the patient flex the wrist 5 times
    c. NMES to the FCR to try and elicit a muscle contraction
    d. Ultrasound to the FCR muscle belly for deep heat

130. A COTA is working with a SCI patient. The COTA is helping teach the patient to use some assistive devices. He is teaching the patient how to use a mouth stick with the computer for typing and for use with an electric wheelchair. He is also showing the patient how to use the electronic page-turner and how to turn pages with the mouth stick for reading. What level SCI would this be appropriate for?
    a. C6
    b. C7
    c. C5
    d. C1-C3

131. A COTA is treating a child who is tactile defensive. All of the following are appropriate treatment activities except for:
    a. Making dough pretzels by kneading and shaping the dough
    b. Using Cheerios or Fruit Loops, string them together to make a necklace
    c. Give the child a brush and have them brush their arms or legs
    D. Using a 1-pound weight, have the child flex and extend his wrist

132. The COTA is treating a patient who is being discharged after a total hip replacement (THR). The COTA is reviewing the discharge plans that the OTR and COTA had collaborated on regarding safety issues in the home. The COTA is cautioning the patient on the type of chairs she should avoid sitting in at home. All of the following should be avoided except for:
    a. Low chairs
    b. Hard chairs
    c. Soft chairs
    d. Reclining chairs

133. The COTA is treating a patient with the diagnosis of rheumatoid arthritis and is making follow-up therapy appointments. What time of day should be avoided when making these appointments because of symptoms of this diagnosis?
    a. Morning
    b. Lunch time
    c. Late afternoon
    d. Dinner time

134. A COTA is working with a patient who has CRPS. This patient sustained a distal radius fracture and developed CRPS two weeks after the injury. The patient has burning pain, pitting edema, and decreased ROM. Which one of the following options would be appropriate treatment techniques?
    a. Gentle ROM, adaptive techniques, patient education, and nerve blocks
    b. Aggressive ROM, adaptive techniques, patient education, and nerve blocks
    c. Static splint to immobilize arm, adaptive techniques, patient education, and nerve blocks
    d. Dynamic wrist splint to increase mobility, adaptive techniques, patient education, and nerve blocks

135. A patient who is hemiplegic has been evaluated by the OTR. The patient is presenting with left-side spasticity with the shoulder in adduction/IR, elbow flexed, forearm pronated, and wrist/fingers flexed. All of the following are appropriate treatment techniques for this patient except for:
    a. PROM using the stretch and hold mobilization technique
    b. Rapid movement stretch to the affected limb
    c. Orthotic positioning to prevent deformity
    d. Neuromuscular electrical stimulation to antagonist muscle group

136. The COTA is treating a patient with left-side spasticity. The patient's shoulder is adducted and IR. The elbow is flexed and the forearm is pronated with the wrist and fingers flexed. All of the following are problems that are associated with this diagnosis except for:
    a. Maceration in the axilla
    b. Problems with dressing such as donning a shirt
    c. Difficulty with PROM of the shoulder that can increase risk of pressure sores
    d. Seizures

137. A COTA is working with a child who has bilateral coordination issues. The child is 7 years old and having difficulty functioning at school with using scissors and performing other bilateral tasks. All of the following are appropriate treatment techniques except for:
    a. Have the child blow bubbles and reach with both hands to pop them
    b. Play with a toy accordion
    c. Tear strips of paper and glue on paper to make a picture
    d. Placing the child's hands in different sensory buckets

138. A COTA is treating a patient in a facility and is working on ROM, strengthening, and balance/coordination activities. The COTA is also working on energy conservation, retraining for ADLs, and safety issues to decrease the risk of falls. What diagnosis would be appropriate for these types of treatment?
    a. Autism
    b. Complex regional pain syndrome
    c. Parkinson disease
    d. Carpel tunnel syndrome

139. All of the following populations would benefit from OT services except for:
    a. People with activity limitations
    b. People with functional impairments
    c. People with cognitive disabilities
    d. People who have language barriers

140. All of the following are facilities where OT services can be provided except for:
    a. Prisons
    b. Inpatient hospital setting
    c. Subacute units
    d. Police stations

141. A COTA is beginning a dressing activity with a child who is 4 years old. What are some things the COTA should be assessing before determining the appropriate treatment activity with the child?
  a. What is the child's cognitive level, how does the child best learn, can the child perform symmetrical tasks
  b. How many peers can the child get along with, how does the child best learn, can the child perform symmetrical tasks
  c. How many siblings does the child have, what is the child's cognitive level, can the child perform symmetrical tasks
  d. Is the child continent, what is the child's cognitive level, how does the child learn best

142. All of the following are different types of dressing equipment for children except for:
  a. Velcro shoe closures
  b. Long-handled shoe horn
  c. Mouth stick
  d. Button hook

143. A COTA is working with a 5-year-old child who presents with decreased FM skills. This child is having difficulty with dressing activities and writing tasks. The COTA needs to work on the child's FM skill to increase independence in these areas. What would some appropriate treatment activities be?
  a. Fastening boards, dress up dolls, and dressing vest
  b. Dressing stick, long-handled shoe horn, and Velcro shoe closure
  c. Tumble forms, reacher, and zipper grip
  d. Sock aid, shoe remover, and button hook

144. What should a COTA do to develop limb and trunk co-contraction patterns for crawling?
  a. Place the child prone in a quadruped position
  b. Place the child in a static standing position
  c. Place the child prone on elbows
  d. Roll the child to side-lying

145. A patient is being treated with modalities to decrease her wrist pain. All of the following are modalities that are used to treat pain except for:
  a. TENS unit
  b. Iontophoresis
  c. Ultrasound
  d. NMES

146. A patient is being treated 1 week after a THR. This patient has the precaution of no hip flexion greater than 90 degrees. What may the COTA suggest that would benefit this patient?
  a. Softer chairs for comfort
  b. Low chairs
  c. Reclining wheelchair
  d. Universal cuff

147. A therapist is working with a spastic patient. He is using rhythmical rotation to help gain ROM with this patient. What treatment technique best describes the therapist's actions:
    a. Active technique used to decrease hypertonia/active motion will increase ROM
    b. Passive technique used to decrease hypertonia/relaxation will increase ROM
    c. Rapid stretch used to decrease hypertonia/stretching will increase ROM
    d. Initiate movement and sustain a contraction through ROM/contractions will increase ROM

148. A patient is being treated after THR. What type of device may be used to reduce the risk of deep vein thrombosis (DVT) for this patient?
    a. Sequential compression device
    b. Knee immobilizer
    c. Balanced suspensions
    d. Reclining wheelchair

149. What type of splint would be best for a patient with carpal tunnel syndrome?
    a. Wrist cock-up in neutral with 3 degrees of ulnar deviation
    b. Wrist cock-up in 30 degrees of wrist flexion
    c. Ulnar gutter splint in 30 degrees of wrist flexion
    d. Radial gutter splint in 30 degrees of wrist flexion

150. A therapist is working with a patient post-CVA who presents with hypertonia. All of the following are appropriate treatment techniques except for:
    a. Slow rocking
    b. Neutral warmth
    c. Deep pressure
    d. Tapping

151. A therapist is treating a patient with Guillain-Barré syndrome. All of the following are appropriate treatment techniques except for:
    a. Sensory re-education activities such as sensory buckets and using sensory sticks to brush affected extremities
    b. A dynamic flexion splint to increase mobility of MCP joints of the hand
    c. Progressive resistive activities such as Theraputty and Velcro board to increase strength in the patient's hands
    d. Cognitive perceptual retraining activities

152. A COTA is treating a patient who has suffered a stroke and a stage 6 in Brunnstrom's stages of motor recovery. Which one of the following would be the most appropriate treatment activity for this patient?
    a. Facilitation of the tonic neck reflex to see motion in the patient's arms
    b. Facilitation of spinal reflexes to result in movement
    c. Resistance applied to contralateral limb to produce movement
    d. Set up three self-care techniques the patient must complete in a certain amount of time

153. A COTA is completing a home evaluation to see if the patient's home is a safe environment for him to be discharged too. This patient uses a wheelchair and the house specifications need to adhere to ADA requirements for doorways, hallways, and countertops. What are the ADA requirements for these specifications?

    a. doorway 30 ", hallway 36", countertops 31"
    b. doorway 32", hallway 36", countertops 31"
    c. doorway 30", hallway 32", countertops 30"
    d. doorway 29", hallway 30", countertops 29"

154. A therapist is treating a person who is in stage 6 of Reisburg's stages of dementia. What would an appropriate treatment activity be?

    a. Have the patient complete a simple self-care task by providing them with verbal cues
    b. Have the patient complete a complex self-care task without cues
    c. Have the patient complete a complex cooking task without cues
    d. Have the patient complete both a self-care and cooking task without cues

155. A patient comes to the clinic with a diagnosis of infraspinatus tear. The patient had surgery 1 week ago to repair the tendon and is instructed to wear a sling at all times by the physician. What AROM do you want to avoid until the tendon is fully healed:

    a. ER
    b. IF
    c. Flexion
    d. Abduction

156. A therapist is working with a 7-year-old child in an outpatient pediatric clinic. The therapist is having the child pull apart Legos with both hands and build a Lego tower. The therapist is also having the child blow bubbles and pop them, alternating with both hands to pop them. What motor issues is this therapist working on?

    a. Sensory processing
    b. Fine motor strength
    c. Gross motor strength
    d. Bilateral coordination

157. A therapist is working with a 5-year-old child in an outpatient pediatric clinic. The child presents with decreased fine motor strength that affects the ability to write. The therapist is having the child perform FM tasks to strengthen the child's hand. The therapist is having the child use clothespins to pick up small items. The therapist is also having the child make a necklace, linking pop beads together. Which one of the following would also be an appropriate treatment activity for this child?

    a. Hiding small objects in Theraputty and having the child pull them out
    b. Have the child catch a ball, throwing it to both the right and left of the child
    c. Finger painting activity
    d. Play with shaving cream

158. An elderly patient is being treated at an outpatient clinic for bilateral hand osteoarthritis. This patient presents with both Heberden and Bouchard nodes on her PIPs and DIPs of bilateral hands. Symptomatically, the patient complains of bilateral hand pain, decreased ROM, and decreased function. All of the following would be appropriate treatment techniques except for:
   a. Heat as-needed for pain
   b. Modifying environment to decrease stress on the joints
   c. Tendon gliding exercises
   d. Aggressive PREs such as Theraputty to increase strength in hand for function

159. A COTA is treating a C6 SCI patient. The patient has all of the following UE motions except for:
   a. Shoulder flexion
   b. Shoulder IR and extension
   c. Wrist flexion
   d. Wrist extension

160. A patient is being discharged to home following a C6 SCI. The patient is using a wheelchair and needs to be able to maneuver around his home environment. What is the minimum doorway clearance needed for the patient to be able to use his wheelchair at home:
   a. 30"
   b. 32"
   c. 26"
   d. 28"

161. All of the following are requirements for NBCOT certification renewal except for:
   a. A completed Certification Renewal Application
   b. Accrual of required Professional Development Units (PDU): 36 PDU in the 3 years between the initial certification date and the renewal due date
   c. Publish 1 article on an area of COTA you are specializing in
   d. Abidance by the NBCOT Candidate/Certificate Code of Conduct

162. What is the COTA's main role in the treatment of Occupational Therapy?
   a. Evaluate patients to determine their POC
   b. Implement treatment with orders from an OTR
   c. Initiate discharge planning
   d. Fabricate both static and dynamic splints independently

163. What does it mean if a COTA's license gets put on probation?
   a. Loss of license for a specific time
   b. Individual needs to meet a condition (more education/supervision, counseling, etc) to get license back
   c. Permanent loss of license
   d. Removal of eligibility for a license

164. What does it mean if the COTA's license gets put on revocation?
   a. Permanent loss of license
   b. Loss of license for a specific time
   c. Individual needs to meet a condition (more education/supervision, counseling, etc) to get license back
   d. A private communication of disapproval of conduct

165. What type of supervision does an entry-level COTA require?
    a. Close supervision by an OTR or supervision by an advanced COTA under supervision of an OTR
    b. Routine supervision by an OTR or supervision by an advanced COTA under supervision of an OTR
    c. Close supervision by an OTR only; COTAs are not allowed to supervise entry-level COTAs
    d. General supervision by an OTR

166. What type of supervision does an intermediate COTA require?
    a. Routine or general supervision by an OTR or advanced COTA under the supervision of an OTR
    b. Close supervision by an OTR or supervision by an advanced COTA under supervision of an OTR
    c. General supervision by an OTR
    d. Routine or general supervision by an OTR only; COTAs are not allowed to supervise intermediate COTAs

167. All of the following are roles of a COTA except for:
    a. Clerical
    b. Prep for new treatment session
    c. Contact Guard during transfers
    d. Evaluate the need for OT services

168. All of the following are principles in the NBCOT Candidate/Certificant Code of Conduct except for:
    a. Certificants shall act in an accurate, truthful, and complete manner in all activities relating to their education, professional work, and research.
    b. Certificants shall not engage in conduct that evidences a lack of knowledge of, or lack of ability to apply, the prevailing principles and /or skills of certified professionals in the field of occupational therapy.
    c. Certificants shall comply with the laws, regulations, and standards governing professional practice in the jurisdictions where they provide occupational therapy services.
    d. Certificants shall promote the profession of OT by publishing articles to aid in the professional development of the profession.

169. All of the following are specific purposes of the American Occupational Therapy Code of Ethics and Ethics Standards except for which one:
    a. Identify and describe the principles supported by the occupational therapy profession
    b. Provide other domains including physical therapy and speech therapy standards in ethical behavior
    c. Assist occupational therapy personnel in recognition and resolution of ethical dilemmas
    d. Socialize occupational therapy personnel to expected standards of conduct

170. The American Occupational Therapy Association (AOTA) Code of Ethics and Standards is a public statement of principles used to maintain a high standard of conduct in the profession. Beneficence is the principle that states all Occupational Therapy personnel shall demonstrate a concern for the well-being and safety of the recipients of their services. All of the following demonstrate this principle except for:
    a. Use all evaluations, planning, intervention techniques, and therapy equipment that are evidence-based and within the recognized scope of occupational therapy practice
    b. Provide Occupational Therapy services that are requested in a timely manner as determined by law, regulation, and policy
    c. Report to an appropriate authority any situations in practice, research, or education that appear unethical or illegal
    d. Avoid inflicting harm to recipients of Occupational Therapy services, employees, students, or research participants

171. The profession of Occupational Therapy identified seven core concepts in the Core Values and Attitudes of Occupational Therapy Practice. Which one of the following is not one of the seven core concepts?
    a. Prudence
    b. Dignity
    c. Freedom
    d. Humility

172. A therapist is treating an open wound at an outpatient OT clinic. Under OSHA regulations for Universal Precautions, what should the therapist's first step be when treating this patient?
    a. Provide a sterile barrier between you and the patient
    b. Make sure the patient is comfortable because open wounds can cause anxiety
    c. Place the patient in mild heat because this can facilitate wound healing
    d. Place the patient in a whirlpool before you see the patient

173. What does an ITP stand for and what population would this be appropriate for?
    a. Individual Therapy Protocol; Geriatrics
    b. Individual Treatment Plan; Birth to 3 years old
    c. Individual Treatment Plan; Geriatrics
    d. Individual Therapy Protocol; Birth to 3 years old

174. All of the following are types of notes except for:
    a. Initial evaluation reports
    b. Re-evaluation notes
    c. Progress notes
    d. Prescription from physician

175. The purpose of a level 1 rotation is to get exposure to different populations in different settings. The students should begin to apply academic knowledge to situations that occur in real life. Which one of the following is the minimum required supervision for this student?
    a. Supervision by an OT practitioner
    b. Supervision by non-OT personnel
    c. No supervision required
    d. Supervision by a COTA

176. What are the three reimbursable service categories to get reimbursement for OT services?
   a. Skilled services, safety concerns, and prevention of secondary complications
   b. Skilled services, vocational concerns, and delaying onset of premorbid conditions
   c. Skilled services, leisure activities, and prevention of secondary complications
   d. Skilled services, social issues, and prevention of secondary complications

177. All of the following are examples of how to correctly document except for:
   a. Use black ink that is waterproof
   b. Sign and date every note
   c. Do not erase
   d. Use correction fluid to correct mistakes

178. A therapist is writing the "O" portion of the SOAP (subjective, objective, assessment, plan) note. Which one of the following best describes what type of information needs to go in this portion of documentation?
   a. Measurable, observable, quantifiable
   b. Measurable, client's perception of treatment, quantifiable
   c. Observable, therapist's perception of treatment, measurable
   d. Quantifiable, observable, client's perception of treatment

179. What does a BIRP note stand for?
   a. Behavior, Intervention, Response, Plan
   b. Behavior, Individual, Response, Plan
   c. Behavior, Individual, Resource, Plan
   d. Behavior, Intervention, Resource, Plan

180. What does a MDS note stand for?
   a. Minimum Data Set
   b. Maximum Data Set
   c. Measureable Data Set
   d. Measureable Dated Series

181. This woman is often termed the "Mother of OT" because she was an early pioneer of the OT profession. She became the director of the OT department for John Hopkins Hospital in 1912 and also helped organize the first professional OT school. In 1922 she established the headquarters of the American Occupational Therapy Association in New York. Who was this woman?
   a. Ruth Brunyate Wiemer
   b. Eleanor Clarke Slagle
   c. Marion Crampton
   d. Mildred Schwagmeyer

182. This woman was an American activist who through a vigorous program of lobbying state legislature and the United States Congress created the first generation of mental asylums. She had found in her home state of Massachusetts how poorly the mentally ill were being treated and lobbied to get them better care. She then went on to found the first public mental hospital in Pennsylvania. Who was this woman?
   a. Dorothea Dix
   b. Eleanor Clark Slagle
   c. Marion Crampton
   d. Mildred Schwagmeyer

183. The Occupational Therapy Code of Ethics and Ethics Standards is a set of principles that are used to guide professional conduct when ethical issues arise. Principle 5 is Procedural Justice. What statement best describes this principle:

    a. This principle is concerned with implementing decisions according to fair processes. Procedures and practices are organized in a fair manner where policies, regulations, and laws are followed.

    b. This principle states that practitioners have a duty to treat the client according to the client's desires and to protect the client's confidential information.

    c. This principle states that practitioners must provide services in a fair and equitable manner.

    d. This principle includes all forms of action that are used to help other people.

184. An OTR is supervising a level 2 student. The OTR is teaching the student how to provide comprehensive, accurate, and objective information when representing the profession. The OTR is teaching the student how to relay accurate and objective information to the patient so that they understand the information. Which principle is the OTR teaching this student according to the Occupational Therapy Code of Ethics and Ethics Standards?

    a. Beneficence

    b. Veracity

    c. Fidelity

    d. Procedural Justice

185. The COTA observes an OTR interrupting a treatment session as another OTR is working on a patient. The OTR is starting an argument about a situation that arose at the company party. What principle according to the Occupational Therapy Code of Ethics and Ethics Standards is the OTR violating?

    a. Fidelity

    b. Social Justice

    c. Procedural Justice

    d. Veracity

186. An OTR is leaving for a few days for vacation. The advanced-level COTA is treating the OTR's established patients according to the documented plan of care. What other duties can the COTA perform while the OTR is away?

    a. Clerical duties

    b. Routine maintenance

    c. Evaluations

    d. Supervise entry-level COTA

187. A COTA was caught giving out a patient's personal data by the supervising OTR. The OTR contacted the state licensing board and the COTA's license was restricted. The COTA had to complete an ethical training course provided by AOTA in order to get his license back. What type of restriction was this COTA's license placed on?

    a. Probation

    b. Suspension

    c. Revocation

    d. Ineligibility

188. An OTR and COTA are doing an on-site visit to a Tyson chicken plant. They are observing the workers and how they complete their jobs. The company wants them to redesign some of their assembly line workstations to decrease the amount of stressed placed on the workers' bodies to prevent injury. What is the correct terminology for what the OTR and COTA are performing?
    a. Ergonomics
    b. Fugue
    c. Service competency
    d. Assessments

189. A therapist has been treating a patient in the clinic for 6 weeks with a diagnosis of postop flexor tendon repair. The patient is seeing the physician next week. The therapist should send all of the following important information to the physician prior to the visit to ensure good communication and quality of care except for:
    a. Objective data
    b. How many times the patient has showed up for visits/how many no shows
    c. Past medical history
    d. The patient's consistency of effort

190. A COTA is treating a patient who has had a stroke. The COTA is implementing the treatment plan that the OTR and the COTA had collaborated on. The patient's status has declined drastically over the past few treatment sessions and the treatment plan is no longer appropriate. What should the COTA's next step be?
    a. Modify treatment plan to fit the patient's current status
    b. Inform the patient's family about the patient's decline
    c. Inform the supervising OTR about the patient's decline
    d. Inform the MD about the patient's decline

191. All of the following are appropriate statements that would go under the "S" component of a SOAP (subjective, objective, assessment, plan) note except for:
    a. The patient reported he has been in a lot of pain over the past few days
    b. The patient did not show up for the appointment
    c. The patient stated he did not wear his splint
    d. The patient said he was feeling depressed

192. A therapist has just gotten a job in an outpatient mental health facility. When working in this type of facility, all of the following are appropriate intervention plans except for:
    a. Stress management groups
    b. Anger management groups
    c. Strength and endurance training
    d. Coping skills group

193. When beginning the intervention process to treat an occupational therapy patient, what is the first step needed in this process:
    a. Referral
    b. Intake note
    c. Progress note
    d. Discharge note

194. What is the definition of "nonskilled" therapy?
   a. Requires professional education and decision-making skills
   b. Maintenance therapy
   c. Safety concerns
   d. Nursing home therapy

195. When documenting for a skilled nursing home, all of the following are appropriate to document except for:
   a. Function of the patient
   b. Safety concerns
   c. Return to home possibility
   d. Individualized treatment plan (ITP)

196. A COTA is treating a pediatric patient to work on his fine motor skills to improve handwriting. The COTA is implementing the treatment plan that both the COTA and OTR collaborated on. The COTA can also do the following duties when treating this child except for:
   a. Initiate discharge planning and discharge child
   b. Set up the treatment room for the child before he arrives
   c. Educate the child's mother on activities the child can do at home to work on FM skills
   d. Schedule the child's follow-up appointments

197. The COTA is expected to adhere to client confidentially regulations when treating patients. All of the following are true when dealing with the concept of client confidentially except for:
   a. Cover up names of patients on a schedule that is open for others to see
   b. Do not discuss the patient's case with unauthorized medical professionals
   c. Do not leave patient's charts on a table where you are treating
   d. Do not arrive late to a patient's scheduled treatment session

198. An OTR is supervising a COTA. The OTR observed the COTA discussing a patient's case with the secretary at lunch. The OTR gave the COTA a reprimand for this behavior. What is the definition of a reprimand?
   a. A private communication between the OTR and COTA regarding the disapproval of conduct
   b. A loss of license for a certain amount of time
   c. A permanent loss of license
   d. Contacting the AOTA to discuss the next step

199. An entry-level COTA is allowed to supervise which of the following medical professionals:
   a. Technicians
   b. Entry-level COTAs
   c. Intermediate COTAs
   d. Level 1 OT fieldwork students

200. An intermediate-level COTA is allowed to supervise which of the following medical professionals:
   a. Intermediate COTA
   b. Level 2 OT fieldwork students
   c. Level 1 OT fieldwork students
   d. Advanced-level OT

Answers and Explanations

1. C: Patients with the diagnosis of Guillain-Barré syndrome usually have muscle weakness and sensory deficits distally, and report pain in their extremities. They do not present with slurred speech. A patient who has suffered a stroke can present with slurred speech. They will have difficulty with a 9-hole peg test and may present with sensory deficits as tested by a Semmes-Weinstein evaluation.

2. D: Myasthenia gravis is characterized by fatigue and muscle weakness, usually in the face and neck. These patients will be able to easily bend over to touch toes. The other answers deal with deficits in the face and neck and are appropriate behaviors when treating a patient with this diagnosis.

3. D: The definition of ideational apraxia is when a patient uses an object incorrectly. These patients do not lack gross or fine motor control. The ability to recognize an object without a visual cue is stereognosis; the inability is astereognosis.

4. A: Brunnstrom's stage 1 of motor recovery is characterized by flaccid limbs and trunk while the nervous system is in a state of inhibition. Therefore, a patient's biceps reflex would not be present. All of the other answers are characteristics of a patient in this stage of motor recovery.

5. D: The COTA is responsible for reporting any change in a patient's status to the supervising OTR so that proper changes can be made in the patient's care. The COTA cannot initiate discharge planning independently without consulting with the OTR. The COTA should not initiate a phone call to the family or to the physician without first consulting with the OTR.

6. D: The correct door swing measurement is 18 inches for a walker

7. A: The correct door swing measurement is 26 inches for a wheelchair

8. C: The ADA requires countertops to be 31 inches high

9. B: Patients with the diagnosis of left CVA present with hesitancy and cautious behavior; therefore, these patients would not initiate a new treatment activity. These patients are overly cautious and may say how hard it is to complete a basic task during their day. They may also not go on a walk alone due to safety fears.

10. D: The symmetric tonic reflex is seen after placing the infant in the crawling position and extending the head. The infant will flex hips and knees and this can be seen when the infant is 4 to 6 months old. The Landau is an upright position of the head. Complete extension of the head, trunk, and extremities is the Landau reflex. The Moro reflex is arm extension in the first phase and the second phase is arm flexion and adduction.

11. B: The Landau reflex occurs in infants 3 to 4 months. This reflex is when the child exhibits complete extension of the head, trunk, and extremities. Birth to 2 months would be the Labyrinthine reflex where the child displays an upright positioning of the head. At 4 to 6 months,

the symmetric tonic reflex is where the child flexes his hips and knees. At 6 to 8 months old, the child displays fewer reflexive behaviors.

12. C: UCL repair, also called gamekeeper's thumb, requires a patient to wear a hand-based thumb spica splint. The precaution of this diagnosis is no lateral deviation until the ligament is fully healed. An FPL repair requires a static flexion splint to the thumb to protect the tendon repair and is forearm based. An EPL repair is a forearm-based static splint to protect the extensor tendon repair. A scaphoid fracture would also involve making a forearm-based splint.

13. C: The role of the COTA is to report any safety issues immediately to the supervising OTR so that they can both address these issues when treating the patient. It is the responsibility of the COTA to always maintain good communication with the supervisory OTR. Once the OTR is communicated with regarding this safety concern, the physician may then be informed of the patient's noncompliance with the splint.

14. D: The supraspinatus muscle controls abduction and flexion of the humerus. It does not play a role in external rotation/internal rotation or extension of the humerus.

15. D: It is important to gather information that is both accurate and reliable. It is not accurate or reliable to gather data from office staff regarding a patient. The other answers provided are all accurate and reliable ways to gather data on a patient.

16. B: The correct anti-deformity position for the wrist and hand is to maintain the wrist at 30-45 degrees of extension with the MPs of the digits flexed to 70 degrees and the thumb IP extended and abducted to prevent further deformity. All of the other positions listed place the hand in a contracted position and will create further deformity.

17. B: Perception deficits are when patients have a disorganized space, difficulty scanning their environment, and often act impulsive. If the patient cannot complete the task because of fine motor/gross motor coordination, then this is a motor issue, not a perceptual issue. A patient who has difficulty with hand-eye coordination has visual spatial perception deficits and some coordination deficits. A patient who cannot recognize objects needed for basic self-care tasks has object agnosia.

18. C: Astereognosis is when patients are unable to determine what everyday objects are with just using tactile properties and no vision. Simultanagnosia is the inability to recognize and interpret an entire visual array at a time. Prosopagnosia is the inability to recognize or identify a known face or individual. Graphesthesia is the inability to identify forms, numbers, and letters written on the skin.

19. D: The Allen Cognitive Level 3 patient will be able determine manual actions and understand tactile cues. He/she is able to repeat the actions of others and understand the relationship between cause and effect. The patient will not, however, be able to follow written instructions. Incorrect answers: Answer A: Level 1: Patients at this level are reflexive with difficulty focusing on external stimuli. They require 24-hour care. Answer B Level 6: Patients plan actions, understand symbolic cues, and can demonstrate problem solving skills. Answer C: Level 5: Patients can understand related cues, demonstrate problem-solving skills, and can complete simple craft activity without written instruction.

20. B: A patient who has ideational apraxia does not know the basic steps that need to be done to complete a task. These patients need physical and verbal prompts in order to complete a basic task

correctly in the correct sequence. Incorrect answers: Dyspraxia is difficulty in planning in regard to movement instead of cognition. This is seen in patients with a diagnosis of cerebral palsy, multiple sclerosis, or Parkinson disease. Akinesia is the inability to initiate movement. Dysmetria is the inability to accurately control the range of movement in muscular acts.

21. B: The protocol for seeing a patient with this diagnosis is usually a few times a week for about 4 to 6 weeks, depending on the patient's progress with decreasing pain and increasing function. After treating a patient with this diagnosis, it is also important to make sure they have a follow-up appointment with the referring physician. Incorrect Answers: Answer A: It would not be appropriate to see a patient 5 times a week with this diagnosis. Answer C: The patient does not dictate how many times a week he is seen. Answer D: It would not be appropriate to provide this patient with an HEP and not see the patient for follow-up visits.

22. C: The patient presents with a diagnosis of FDP/FDS repair 2 days postop. The precaution for this diagnosis is active motion, which will rupture the repair of the tendon. As a clinician during this stage of postop care, you are responsible to check for edema/swelling of affected area and to watch the wound for signs of infection. You are also responsible for PROM of all the digits because AROM is contraindicated at this point in the healing process to maintain joint mobility.

23. D: A static splint does not have any moving parts and is used to prevent the patient from moving an affected joint. These splints also help to align the joints for healing and reducing pain. A dynamic splint is a splint where moving parts are included to help with various ROM issues.

24. B: The Kohlman Evaluation of Living Skills and Allen Cognitive Levels are used for functional assessments and the Jacobs Prevocational Assessment is used for a work assessment. The Schroeder-Block-Campbell can be used for both SI patients and for functional assessments as well.

25. C: Social skills are not in the KELS 5 areas of living skills assessment.

26. B: Answers A and D do not have the COTA collaborating with the supervising OTR for completing steps of the assessment, and answer C involves the physician, which is not needed when giving a patient an assessment.

27. C: Allen Cognitive Levels Screen is an example of an interview-style assessment. The assessment involves having patients complete a running stitch activity to help determine their cognitive level. Rating Scale Activity Configuration/Prevocational Inventory/Sensorimotor History are all examples of interview-style assessments in which patients are being interviewed by the clinician to find out their particular skill level.

28. C: A COTA's role when giving assessments is making sure he/she is at all times collaborating with the OTR during the process. Therefore, when the COTA scores and interprets results, he/she must do so in conjunction with the OTR and not act alone during this process.

29. A: A C7 SC injured patient has the triceps, extrinsic finger extensors, and flexor carpi radialis fully innervated. SCI injured patients with C6 last innervated muscles do not include wrist flexors or digital muscles. C5 levels have shoulder muscles and biceps last innervated and C4 levels have respiration and scapula elevation innervated.

30. B: The patient with a C5 SC injury has elbow flexion and supination, shoulder external rotation and shoulder abduction to 90. These patients also are able to use gravity to provide shoulder

adduction, pronation, and IR. Therefore, these patients are able to use the adaptive equipment provided in the question to function.

31. D: The definition of MMT muscle grade 0 is no muscle contraction is seen or felt. A grade 2 or higher would mean the patient presents with ROM of these affected muscles.

32. D: The definition of MMT grade 2+ is when the patient is able to move 50% of the full ROM against gravity or full ROM with gravity eliminated, applying slight resistance. MMT grade 3 is answer A; MMT grade 2- is answer B; MMT grade 3- is answer C.

33. B: A MMT grade of 3+ is also known as Fair Plus. Incorrect answers: Answer A: Grade 3 is when a patient can move through part of ROM against gravity/no resistance. Answer C: Patient can move partially through ROM against gravity with moderate resistance. Answer D: Patient can move through full ROM with moderate resistance.

34. B: A patient with a Rancho Level 4 may be confused and agitated and may display inappropriate behavior. They need maximum assist and have a short attention span. Incorrect answers: Answer A is level 5, which is not agitated. Answer C is level 1. Answer D is level 3

35. B: The adult standard wheelchair dimensions are width of 18 inches/depth of 16/height of 20.

36. A: Wheelchair ramps should have a 1" vertical rise for every 12" of horizontal distance.

37. D: A patient with this diagnosis is not allowed to flex his hip past 90, perform IR/ER or adduction/cross legs. No extension is not a precaution of this diagnosis.

38. C: An individualized education plan (IEP) is performed in a school setting for children ages 3-18 years, with emphasis on education for that child. These are not performed in a hospital setting.

39. C: The O portion of the note should not include how the clinician assessed the treatment. That portion of the note should go under A. The Objective/O part of the note includes parts of the treatment that are measureable, quantifiable, and observable. Therefore, answer C is part of the Assessment part of the note as it is more of a subjective view/assessment of how the therapist thought the patient performed in treatment that day.

40. A: The palmer-supinated grasp is when a child of 1 to 1½ years old grips the pencil with power on the ulnar side of their hand and writes on the paper as their arm and hand move. The incorrect answers: Digital-pronated grasp is when a child holds the pencil with her fingers/wrist in neutral with slight ulnar deviation/forearm pronated. Arm moves as a unit. Static tripod grasp is when the child grasps the pencil proximally with continuous adjustments by other hand, no fine localized movements. Dynamic tripod grasp is when the child grasps the pencil with precise opposition/MCP joints stabilized during fine localized movements of PIP joints.

41. D: This patient needs to be placed in an elbow brace that prevents full flexion of the elbow, which will increase the pressure on the ulnar nerve in the elbow. These symptoms are often increased at night when a person is sleeping because most people sleep with their elbows flexed.

42. C: When patients have an ulnar nerve injury, they often present with hyperextension of the ring/pinky MCPs because of intrinsic muscle imbalance. Answer A is flexion of the PIP joint with

hyperextension of the DIP joints. Answer B is hyperextension of the PIP joint with flexion of the DIP joint. Answer D involves the thumb, index, and middle digits.

43. B: The inability to identify body parts on self or someone else is called Autotopagnosia. The inability to identify forms, numbers, and letters written on the skin is Graphesthesia.

44. A: Central Cord Syndrome is injury to the central cord, which often occurs from hyperextension injuries. Patients have more UE loss then LE deficits. Answer B describes Brown-Sequard Syndrome. Answer C describes Anterior Cord Syndrome. Answer D describes Conus Medullaris Syndrome.

45. A: A patient with this high level of SCI has limited movement of their neck and head and needs assistive devices to do basic skills. These patients also cannot breathe on their own. Answers B-D all involve a certain amount of motor control that a SCI of this level will not display.

46. B: The COTA is not allowed to perform an evaluation to determine if OT services are needed and must reschedule the evaluation for the OTR to perform. Answers A/C/D all involve having the COTA perform the evaluation independent of the OTR, which is not allowed within a COTA's guidelines.

47. A: The COTA's role in discharge planning is to be able to communicate the discharge plans to the patient and the patient's family. The COTA needs to make sure everyone understands the HEP for home follow-through and is able to review all safety guidelines to make a safe, smooth transition for everyone involved.

48. D: A patient with a CHF level 4 often has pain, palpitations, or angina at rest and during all physical activities, even low-level activities. Answer A describes a CHF level 2, where the patient has slight limitations during physical activity. Answer B describes a CHF level 1, where a patient is not limited by pain, palpations, angina, etc. Answer C describes a level 3 CHF patient. This patient is limited by physical activity and also during less than normal activity when experiencing symptoms.

49. C: A patient will can present with pain, tingling, and numbness of the thumb, index, and middle with the diagnosis of CT. These symptoms are often increased at night when a patient flexes his wrists to sleep or uses a computer with poor workstation design. Radial tunnel syndrome occurs when the radial nerve is compressed. They symptoms include tenderness at the lateral epicondyle and pain when the wrist is extended. Cubital tunnel syndrome is when the ulnar nerve is compressed at the elbow and the ring and pinky are affected in the hand. De Quervain syndrome is a tendonitis of the thumb involving the extensor pollicis brevis and abductor pollicis longus muscles.

50. D: Autotopagnosia is a patient's inability to identify body parts on self or someone else. Prosopagnosia is the inability to recognize or identify a known face or individual. Simultanagnosia is the inability to recognize and interpret an entire visual array at a time. Graphesthesia is the ability to identify forms, numbers, and letters written on the skin.

51. A: WFL stands for within functional limits. This means a patient's ROM is allowing her to perform all their functional tasks. This does not have anything do to with a fracture status and the "L" stands for limits not level.

52. B: The SOAP note is a documentation method used commonly in rehab situations. It requires making a subjective observation, an objective observation, an assessment of what is wrong, and a plan to correct it.

53. D: A patient's health record should be specific to the current diagnosis under which the patient is being treated for. This record should include what services the patient has received and how the patient has responded to treatment. This health record should not include a prior vocational assessment from a past employer as it does not pertain to the current diagnosis.

54. B: Muscle twitching is not a side effect of tricyclic antidepressants. Postural hypotension, seizures, and urinary retention are all side effects of tricyclic antidepressants.

55. B: The following are side effects of MAOIs: sweating, palpations, headache, increase in BP, postural hypotension, vomiting/nausea, drowsiness, and weakness. These patients would not present with constipation issues or slurred speech. They would not present with urinary retention or tremors/shivering.

56. D: A patient with this diagnosis will take on another person's identity. This diagnosis is not associated with restricted emotion/decreased speech and cognitive ability or inability to socialize in group setting. These patients will exhibit behaviors of another person instead of behaviors of themselves.

57. B: Swan neck deformity is when a patient presents with hyperextension of the PIP and flexion of the DIP. Boutonniere deformity is flexion of the PIP and hyperextension of the DIP. Osteoarthritis is characterized by nodes at the lateral borders of the joints and RA deformity is characterized by swelling and zig-zag deformity of the hands with radial drift of the wrist and ulnar drift of the digits.

58. A: The COPM is an assessment that is used with all populations in a variety of developments stages and disabilities. It looks at a patient's self-care, productivity, and leisure skills. This assessment does not look at a patient's vocational skills/social skills/or ROM status.

59. B: The Biomechanical FOR is used with patients who present with limitations in movement, inadequate muscle strength, and loss of endurance in occupations. A Motor Skills Acquisition is used with a pediatric population. A Psychodynamic and Role Acquisition is used with a mental health population under psychosocial frameworks.

60. C: Vocational performance is not an example of a performance skill. Performance skills are sensory perception skills/motor and praxis skills/emotional regulation skills/cognitive skills/communication skills/social skills.

61. C: The COTA's responsibility is to report any change of behavior observed with a patient to the supervising OTR so that modifications can be made in the patient's care. The COTA and OTR can then collaborate together on what changes need to be made to the POC to ensure the safety of the patient.

62. D: A COTA is not allowed to independently administer an evaluation. He can contribute to an evaluation but cannot do it independently. The COTA can, however, work as a practitioner, teacher, and peer educator.

63. B: A patient with a C5 SCI last fully innervated level and key muscles are biceps, brachialis, brachioradialis, supinator, infraspinatus, and deltoid. Therefore, they would need moderate assistance with their UE and maximum assistance with their LE. These patients would not need max assist for both as they do have function of their elbow flexors and certain shoulder muscles. They would need more than minimal assistance for their UE and more than mod assist with their LE. Therefore, the other answers would not work.

64. A: A patient with a diagnosis of SCI C1-C3 can chew, swallow, talk and blow. These patients are on a ventilator and would not be able to operate a wheelchair or perform self-care activities with minimal assistance. They do not have the muscle innervation to complete tasks with answers B-D.

65. B: The palmer grasp is typically seen in children who are 5 months old. A child who is 4 months old will display the primitive squeeze grasp where the thumb in not involved. A child who is 8 months old will display the radial digital grasp where the object is held with the opposed thumb and fingertips. A child who is 6 months old will have the radial palmer grasp where the fingers on the far side of the object press it against the thumb on the radial side of the hand with the wrist flexed.

66. C: When a patient is being treated for an infection in a hand clinic, this patient often will need to be seen 5 times per week until the infection in under control. Wounds can change quickly within a 24-hour period and an open infection will need to be closely monitored. If a patient is having a lot of pain, she needs to report to the physician to rule out an infection instead of being seen by a therapist 5 times a week. Insurance is not going to pay for a nervous patient who wants to be seen instead of what the proper protocol for the diagnosis is. You would also not see a patient 5 times per week because she is not compliant with her HEP.

67. B: The Kleinert protocol for flexion tendon injuries states that at 0-4 weeks postop, the therapist should initiate passive flexion and active extension exercises within the confines of the splint. The patient should be in a dorsal block splint with the MPs at 60-70 degrees/IPs 0 degrees, allowing for passive flexion and active extension exercises using rubber-band traction. The Duran protocol is where a patient passively flexes all the digits into the palm without performing active extension exercises. Active ROM is contraindicated at this point in treatment as it will rupture the tendon and ruin the repair, requiring further surgery for the patient. The answer of passive flexion and passive extension does not indicate the Kleinert protocol.

68. B: Patients with Oculomotor Deficits present with saccadic eye movement, difficulty with tracking, convergence and divergence, and diplopia. They have difficulty with hand-eye coordination, reading, cutting, and pouring activities.

69. A: Astereognosis is the inability to identify objects with vision occluded. Therefore, A would be the appropriate answer. This definition does not deal with having the patient write down characteristics of self or involve FM/GM tasks. A treatment activity of having the patient look at the object would not be working on the diagnosis of astereognosis because the patient is allowed to see the object.

70. C: Patients with a C4 SCI have scapular elevation and the ability to breathe on their own. They are able to use a long straw with a straw holder but do not have to ability to use any of the other adaptive equipment. Those items are used for a C5 SCI patient. A level C5 has the muscle innervation of the biceps, brachialis, brachioradialis, supinator, infraspinatus, and deltoid.

Therefore, that patient can use a wrist splint with a universal cuff, suspension sling, and ratchet splint.

71. C: This patient can benefit from sensory buckets to try and increase sensation in the right hand. The use of modalities such as ultrasound and hot pack is contraindicated with a patient who has this diagnosis. Electrical stimulation or a resting hand splint does not address the patient's sensation issues.

72. C: A patient who presents with a hypersensitive scar would benefit from sensory buckets to apply sensory stimulation to the hypersensitive scar. This treatment activity will work to stop the sensory endings from over-firing, which can be the cause of a hypersensitive scar. Iontophoresis using dexamethasone is used for inflammatory conditions and ultrasound as a heat modality is used for increasing ROM. A wrist brace to protect the scar would not help to decrease the hypersensitivity as it would not allow the scar to come into contact with any sensory stimulation, which would help to calm down the scar.

73. C: A patient who has a MET level of 1.4-2 should perform all functional activities while sitting. A patient with a MET level of 2 or higher can begin to perform activities while standing

74. B: The patient who has Dupuytren disease will need a postop splint to maintain all digits in extension. These patients will be instructed to wear the splint at all times, often for 2 weeks. You would not want to flex the MPs to 70 degrees in the splint as this would place the hand in a contracted state, which is what the surgery for Dupuytren is correcting. These patients most always need a splint postop to correct the flexion deformity that is associated with Dupuytren disease; therefore, the last two answers are inappropriate.

75. D: A 6- to 7-month-old child should be able to self-feed with a cracker. The activity of picking up Cheerios will work on the patient's fine motor skills. Having the child eat the Cheerios will help with increasing independence with feeding goals. A child who is 9 months old will be able to drink from a cup and will be able to hold and bang a spoon on the table. A child who is 12 to 14 months old will be able to bring a spoon to mouth with food but often times will spill it until they reach the age of 18 months, when this developmental milestone becomes more successful.

76. B: A child at 4 months of age should be able to place their hands together at midline when trying to reach for a toy. A child of this age will not be able to sit unassisted because of decreased truck stability, and the radial and pincer grasps are not present in a child at this age.

77. D: A patient with a C6 SCI does not need a long-handled straw. They are able to use a cup with larger handles in order to drink independently. They can use a universal cuff at this level along with a rocker knife and a cup with long handles. These patients have shoulder flexion, shoulder internal/extension/adduction, pronation, and wrist tenodesis.

78. B: If a patient leans too forward in a wheelchair, the armrests are too low. If their shoulders are elevated, the armrests are too high. A patient leaning forward has nothing to do with footrest height.

79. B: An MMT of 3+ FCR would indicate a patient is able to move through complete ROM against gravity with slight resistance. Therefore, having a patient pick up cones against gravity would provide the patient with minimal resistance and work to increase this MMT level. If the patient is picking up cones in a gravity-eliminated plane, this activity would be too easy for this patient. If the

activity was to do 3 lb wrist curls against gravity, this would be too hard and would overfatigue the patient's already weak muscles. NMES would not be used in a gravity-eliminated plane to facilitate ROM because the patient is already able to do this without the modality.

80. A: If the COTA removed the doorstops to all the doors, ¾ inches would be added to the width of the door, so the wheelchair could safely pass through at 32¼ inches. 32 inches is the minimum width a wheelchair can go through a doorway. All of the other answers are incorrect because they would not increase the door width so that the wheelchair can safely go through.

81. D: The most appropriate answer is D because the COTA should place the objects out of order to see if the patient can still complete the task. Verbal and written instructions would not be the best choice when grading this activity because the patient can already complete the activity without them. Having the patient try to find the objects is too complex. It would be better to rearrange the objects to see if the patient can complete the task before removing the objects from the patient's vision.

82. B: Answer A is 4-5 MET level/ Answer C is 6-7 MET level/ Answer D 7-8 MET level

83. D: Autonomic dysreflexia is a potential life-threatening situation for SCI patients and requires immediate attention. These patients experience high blood pressure, headaches, sweating, bradycardia, and anxiety. Because it can be a life-threatening situation, the COTA needs to call for immediate medical assistance. The COTA does not have time to report to the OTR supervisor during this critical situation. The COTA would not lay the patient down or have the patient place his arms overhead. This patient needs medical assistance from a medical professional who is qualified to handle this immediate situation.

84. B: SCI patients are not a higher risk of RA. SCI patients are at a higher risk of osteoporosis, pressure ulcers, and thermal dysregulation.

85. B: Central Cord Syndrome is an injury to the central cord resulting from hyperextension injuries. Typically, these patients have more UE deficits than LE; therefore, B would be the best answer. These patients could benefit from using an UE arm bike, working on fine motor skills with the 9-hole peg test, and working on both gross and fine motor skills with a cone activity. The other answers involve activities for the patient's lower extremity, which is not as affected with Central Cord Syndrome.

86. D: Answers A-C are all ways to increase a patient's independence with dressing tasks when FM/GM deficits are present. The use of oversized shirts and dresses makes it easier for a patient with limited mobility to dress. Pants and skirts with elastic waistbands eliminate the need to button or zipper, which will increase independence despite a lack of fine motor control. A long-handled shoe horn will help a patient put on shoes despite decreased gross motor control. A C-bar splint is used to decrease thenar eminence stiffness/deformity of the hand and would not aid in dressing tasks.

87. A: A patient with Parkinson disease would benefit from UE/LE ROM, strengthening exercises, energy conservation techniques, and safety modifications. In option B/C, a patient does not need anger management or time management groups. In answer D, sensory integration is not appropriate with this population.

88. C: Crawling is a very important developmental milestone because it helps develop arches in the hands, which helps with FM skills such as handwriting. Crawling also provides weightbearing opportunities that aid with shoulder stability. Learning the alphabet and numbers for infants birth to 12 months of age is too advanced. Finger painting may be fun but would not be considered a developmental milestone.

89. C: Answers A, B, and D are all activities that are appropriate for children 2 to 3 years of age when working on prewriting skills. Tracing over letters would be an appropriate activity for a child who is 5 to 6.

90. C: Children who are tactile defensive do not like surprises, so coming up behind the child would startle him or make him upset. It is always better to approach these children from the front. These children also do not respond well to light touch and prefer a firm touch to compensate for being tactile defensive.

91. D: The 9-hole peg test is for patients who have decreased FM skills. This is not a characteristic of a child with tactile defensiveness. The other treatment activities are activities that a child with tactile defensiveness would benefit from.

92. D: It would not be appropriate to place the child near the auditory source; this would upset the child. She may become distractible and not be able to function in her classroom when placed by the auditory source. This would decrease the child's ability to function well in her environment. Using earplugs for school and placing the child away from the auditory source are good ways to modify the environment for a child with this diagnosis. Preparing the child ahead of time for the sounds she may hear will help her cope better with the environmental sounds.

93. D: It is contraindicated to place the adverse texture in the child's mouth. The COTA's job is to desensitize the child to certain textures so that eventually she can tolerate different food textures. Placing the adverse food directly into the child's mouth without desensitizing her will upset her and not improve the issue. By finger painting with different food and textures, a fun environment is created for the child to get used to different textures. Providing external stimuli to the child's face and mouth gets the child desensitized before trying new textures in her mouth. The blowing through a straw activity is creating fun by using a game that involves a mouth activity to help with oral-motor desensitization techniques.

94. B: A child would not benefit from an anger management group. The underlying issue is sensory and those are the areas that need to be addressed in treatment. A child 5 years old or younger needs to be taught coping skills to use when feeling restless in his environment. This could be teaching the child to squeeze a ball when these feeling arise. These children can also benefit from sensory stimulation to calm down these behaviors, such as slow rocking in a chair or being wrapped up in a blanket.

95. D: A-C are all treatment activities that will increase the child's fine motor strength to increase endurance to perform writing tasks. Answer D may help by modifying the pencil but will not increase the child's FM strength.

96. C: The best way to position a patient at their workstation is with hips/knees/elbows all at 90 degrees. This is a basic principle when designing a patient's workstation ergonomically.

97. A: A precaution of using ultrasound is over metal implants. It is safe to use over the dorsal and volar surface of the wrist as long as it is not directly over the metal implants. A supinator muscle is also safe to ultrasound.

98. C: A patient with muscular dystrophy is experiencing a gradual weakening of their skeletal muscles. These patients can benefit from FM/GM tasks and adaptive techniques. These patients do not receive nerve blocks for pain. A complex regional pain syndrome patient who is experiencing burning, consistent pain would benefit from a nerve block.

99. D: Client factors are beliefs, characteristics, and abilities of the patient. They are not beliefs of the patient's family; therefore, the COTA would not them into consideration when writing the goals.

100. C: When treating a patient with CRPS, it is contraindicated to perform PROM/aggressive ROM exercises because these may increase the symptoms of the diagnosis. Strengthening exercises are also contraindicated. These patients benefit from gentle ROM as tolerated, modalities as needed, edema control techniques, adaptive techniques, and patient education until symptoms are reduced.

101. D: A dynamic extension splint is used for patients who have a radial nerve injury, which affects the patient's wrist and finger extensors. A patient who has an ulnar nerve injury can benefit from a wrist splint positioned at 30 degrees of flexion if the ulnar nerve injury is a low lesion. If the ulnar nerve injury is a high lesion, the elbow would be included. The MCP flexion block splint is often used with ulnar nerve patients who have an intrinsic muscle imbalance and present with hyperextension of the MCPs of the ring and pinky fingers.

102. A: A dorsal wrist splint in neutral would not be appropriate for a median nerve lacerated patient. The wrist needs to be positioned in 30 degrees of flexion to protect the median nerve repair and allow it to heal. A wrist splint in neutral is more appropriate for a patient with carpel tunnel syndrome. A patient who has a median nerve laceration can benefit from a wrist and elbow splint positioned in flexion, depending on if the laceration is a low or high lesion. A C-bar splint is also often used with a median nerve injury to prevent adduction contractures.

103. C: The purpose of a serial splint is to achieve a slow, progressive increase in a patient's ROM by continuously remolding the splint as the patient's ROM increases. These splints can be static or dynamic and the patient is instructed to wear the splints for a long period of time throughout the day with a small amount of tension applied to the joint. When the patient's joint mobility increases to a nonstretch status within the splint, it is modified slightly to increase tension and worn for a long period of time. Answer A and D would not work because they have the patient wearing the splint for a short amount of time, and Answer B would not be appropriate because it maintains the joint with the same tension in the splint.

104. D: A wrist cock-up splint is a static wrist splint that allows for full ROM of all the fingers. It is often used to treat carpal tunnel (CT) patients by placing the wrist in a neutral position to decrease CT pressure and reduce CT symptoms. It also is used in patients who have wrist pain to rest the painful wrist, as seen in patients who have acute RA. A person who presents with claw deformity has hyperextension of the ring and pinky MCPs, which a wrist cock-up splint would not be appropriate for.

105. A: Slow rolling/rocking is effective when treating a patient who has hypertonicity or spasticity. This is an inhibitory technique that can decrease spasticity. Fast rocking for this type of patient is contraindicated because it often can increase a patient's spasticity. Neck co-contraction is facilitated

when the goal is head and neck control and noxious stimulation is sometimes used as a facilitatory technique to help normalize flaccid muscles.

106. D: Slow stroking is an inhibitory technique used for patients who have overactive muscles/spastic muscles. You would not want to use an inhibitory technique when treating a patient with low tone or flaccid muscles. Facilitatory techniques such as tapping, noxious odor, painful stimuli, quick stretch, light rapid brushing, and heavy joint compression would be beneficial to this patient.

107. A: Heavy joint compression is a facilitatory technique used with patients with flaccid/low tone muscles. Pleasant odor is an inhibitory technique that helps to normalize hypertonic/spastic muscles. Slow rocking/slow rolling is also an inhibitory technique that is used to relax overactive or spastic muscles.

108. D: A patient who is diagnosed with severe dementia is often hostile and uncooperative. These patients have safety issues such as falling down and wandering, which need to be addressed. They do not present with seizures or other medical conditions unless they have a dual diagnosis. A patient with dementia alone should not present with the increased potential for having a seizure.

109. C: When giving an assessment, the COTA is allowed to organize the information and collaborate with the OTR on the information. The COTA can document the assessment and write down what he sees through observation, interviews, and chart reviews. The COTA, however, cannot organize, analyze, and interpret the results independently from the OTR. He can aid in this collaboration but is not allowed to do it on his own.

110. D: The Glasgow Coma Scale on best verbal response is as follows: 1 = no sound; 2 = incomprehensible; 3 = inappropriate words; 4 = confused; 5 = oriented.

111. B: According to the Glasgow Coma Scale, the following numbers represent the best eye response behavior of a coma patient: 1 = no eye opening; 2 = eye opening in response to pain; 3 = eye opening to speech; 4 = eye opening spontaneously.

112. C: If a patient has akathisia, he is unable to remain calm. These patients often exhibit anxiety and are unable to remain still. These patients benefit most in treatment if the environment is calm and relaxing, without a lot of external stimulation that may increase their anxiety. If the COTA tried to treat this patient in a loud cafeteria or in group treatments with a lot of people, this may increase the patient's anxiety and inhibit his ability to perform treatment activities.

113. B: Echopraxia is when a patient displays behaviors by repetitive imitation of another person's movements. Ideational apraxia is when a patient uses a common object incorrectly. Prosopagnosia is when a person is unable to identify a person well known. Anosognosia is when a person is unaware of their deficits.

114. A: Color agnosia is the patient's inability to remember or recognize different colors. By holding up different colored flashcards and having the patient name the color, you are working on associating a color to the name of the color. By having the patient use crayons and reading what color needs to go where when coloring a paper, you are again using an associative technique to match the color with its name. By having the patient organize the blocks by color and naming what color group each one is, you are again associating the color with its name. If you simply have the

patient organize the color blocks together without stating the color groups, you are not working on learning on the colors and their names.

115. B: A patient who is characterized as a level 3 in the Allen Cognitive Level Test is able to determine what manual actions are needed for a simple task, so answer C is appropriate. This patient is also able to repeat the actions of others and can follow a task if it is demonstrated, so answers A and D would be appropriate. A patient in this level is not able to follow written directions. A patient who can follow written instructions would be characterized as a level 4 in the Allen Cognitive Level Test.

116. A: The definition of a task-oriented group is when the goal is to increase the members' knowledge of feelings, thoughts, and values through the process of a task-oriented activity with other group members. The definition of a topical group is to increase the member's activity performance through problem solving and this is a verbal-based group. The definition of instrumental group is when the goal of the group is to have the members function at the highest level of their ability for as long as possible. This is used in populations who have chronic disabilities. The goal of a thematic group is to assist members in acquiring the knowledge and attitudes for a specific set of skills.

117. B: The goal of a topical is to improve the member's activity performance through problem solving. This is a verbal based group where the focus is to have the members verbalize what activities they are involved in and what steps need to be done to complete the task. A task oriented group's goal is to increase a member's awareness of feelings, thoughts, and values through task oriented activities. An instrumental group works on having its members function at their highest functional level for an extended period of time. A Thematic group is working towards having its members learn the knowledge for a specific set of skills independently.

118. D: A resting hand splint is a static wrist-hand orthosis used to immobilize a patient's wrist and hand to prevent deformity. The MCPs and IPs are maintained in a lengthened position to prevent any joint contractures. This type of splint is not used to increase wrist or hand joint mobility.

119. D: De Quervain disease is an inflammation of the extensor pollicis brevis and abductor pollicis longus muscles. These muscles allow the thumb to radially abduct. The correct position to allow these tendons to heal is with the wrist positioned in slight extension with the thumb included. A wrist cock-up splint does not include the thumb and would not help. A C-bar splint is used for medial nerve injuries and is hand-based. A thumb spica with the wrist positioned in slight flexion would put tension on these tendons, so it would be contraindicated.

120. D: A child who is 3½ years of age should be able to manipulate scissors in a forward motion and be able to coordinate the lateral direction of the scissors. She should be able to cut paper in a straight line and cut out simple geometric shapes. A child of this age will not be able to cut out complex shapes. This is usually seen with a 6- to 7-year-old child. Therefore, the activity would be too hard for a child who is 3½ years old.

121. C: A patient with a MET level of 1.4-2 will perform all functional tasks while sitting. He can walk across a room at a slow pace, with carefully monitoring for overfatigue. At this level, no isometrics are allowed and are contraindicated for this patient.

122. B: The symmetric tonic reflex is present in children 4 to 6 months of age. When in a prone position and their head is extended, you will see the hips and knees flex. The Landau reflex is seen

in children 3 to 4 months of age, when the child is placed in a horizontal prone suspension and you see complete extension of the child's extremities. The Labyrinthine righting reflex is seen with children from birth to 2 months. This is seen by holding the infant vertically and tilting slowly in different directions; the child will maintain an upright position of their head. The Moro reflex can be seen at birth and occurs when the child's head is rapidly dropped backwards. The child will extend arms straight out at the sides at right angles to the body with the body arched and head extended. This is a protective response.

123. C: A skier's thumb diagnosis is a rupture of the ulnar collateral ligament of the MCP joint in the thumb. A hand-based thumb spica would protect this ligament until it was able to heal. A wrist cock-up or a MP block would not include the thumb and would provide no protection. A forearm-based thumb spica would not be needed as the ligament does not articulate with the wrist.

124. B: The Labyrinthine righting reflex orients the head in space/maintains face vertical. The Landau reflex breaks up flexor dominance. The Moro reflex is a protective response when a child's head is dropped backwards. The Galant reflex facilitates trunk stabilization.

125. B: After a patient undergoes rotator cuff surgery to repair the tendon, it is contraindicated to do any AROM/AAROM to the planes of motion that the tendon is involved in. The supraspinatus tendon performs shoulder abduction and flexion, so A/AAROM of these planes at 7 days postop may ruin the repair. If you performed no ROM to the shoulder joint following a repair, the patient would most likely end up with a frozen shoulder. An appropriate treatment protocol would be PROM of all shoulder planes of motions to maintain the joint integrity while protecting the repair at the same time.

126. A: A patient with contrast sensitivity deficits has difficulty recognizing faces, distinguishing colors, and stumbles frequently. These patients can benefit from environmental adaptations such as changing color to increase contrast, decreasing patterns, and reducing clutter. By blending color, increasing patterns, and increasing clutter, the environment would be more difficult for these patients. Eye movement activities, visu-motor tasks, and scanning tasks are appropriate for a patient with oculomotor deficits. Scanning training, safety adaptations, and increased lighting in rooms are appropriate for patients with peripheral visual deficits.

127. A: A patient who has oculomotor deficits will present with saccadic eye movements, difficulty with tracking, decreased ROM, and diplopia. They have hand-eye coordination issues, difficultly with mobility, reading, cutting, and pouring. Therefore, visuomotor tasks, eye movement activities, and scanning tasks would be appropriate. A patient with peripheral visual deficits will benefit from larger print, yellow and amber sunglasses, and increased lighting in the room. A patient who has visual acuity deficits will benefit from magnification, larger print, and community resources. A patient who has contrast sensitivity deficits will benefit from changing color to increase contrast, decreasing patterns, and reducing clutter.

128. C: An MMT muscle grade of the ECRL/ECRB indicates that the patient is unable to complete full ROM of wrist extension in a gravity-eliminated plane. This is without any resistance, so in a gravity-eliminated plane, picking up soup cans would be too hard for this patient. Any activity against gravity would be too hard for this patient until the patient can complete full ROM of the wrist in a gravity-eliminated plane.

129. C: An MMT grade of 0 for the FCR indicates that a contraction of the muscle can be palpated but there is no motion noted. Therefore, answers A and B would not make sense because the patient is unable to flex the wrist at all. Ultrasound for deep heat will not increase or work towards

increasing a patient's mobility. Neuromuscular electrical stimulation (NMES) can help stimulate a stronger action potential within the muscle to try and gain some motion.

130. D: A patient with a level C1-C3 can chew, swallow, talk, and blow; therefore, she has the ability to use a mouth stick for certain tasks to increase function. A SCI level of C5 or higher has the ability to use their arms because at the C5 level, biceps, brachialis, brachioradialis, supinator, infraspinatus, and deltoids are present. Therefore, they would not need a mouth stick for certain functional tasks. These patients benefit from the use of certain splints as a universal cuff to help them function.

131. D: A child who is tactile defensive feels that a particular sensation is noxious or uncomfortable. The treatment for this type of disorder is to gently introduce different textures or sensations to the child to get her used to different sensory stimulation. Kneading dough and making dough pretzels provides sensory input in a fun way for this child. The same concept occurs with making food necklaces. Another technique is having the child brush her arms and legs to get used to that type of sensory stimulation without it feeling uncomfortable. Using a 1 lb weight and having the child flex/extend their wrist works on strengthening and is not a sensory technique.

132. B: After a patient has had a THR, she will have trouble getting out of chairs because of pain that is associated with a THR. Low chairs, soft chairs, and chairs that recline are all more difficult to get up from than a hard chair. A hard chair should be avoided.

133. A: With a diagnosis of RA, most patients have a difficult time starting their day because of pain and stiffness of their joints when they get out of bed in the morning. These patients often need time to heat up their joints and stretch them out before they can do self-care tasks such as dressing and brushing teeth. Therefore, morning appointments should be avoided with this population.

134. A: A patient with CRPS will benefit from gentle ROM, adaptive techniques, patient education, and nerve blocks. These treatment techniques will help the patient control the pain and increase their ROM for functional use. Aggressive ROM is contraindicated in this patient because it can increase the symptoms of the diagnosis. Static splints to immobilize the joint will increase stiffness in the patient and dynamic splints will increase the symptoms.

135. B: A patient who presents with spasticity on one side of the body will benefit from a slow passive stretch to the extremity. This will help inhibit spasticity and allow the extremity to gain more motion. A rapid movement to the affected limb can increase the stretch reflex and result in a sudden increase in muscle tone. Orthotic positioning such as a resting hand splint will position the hand in a lengthened position, preventing deformity. Neuromuscular stimulation to the antagonist muscle groups will help facilitate joint motion in the affected limb. When you stimulate the antagonist muscle, it will cause the agonist muscle to relax and increase ROM.

136. D: A patient with left-side spasticity is at risk for maceration of the skin in the axilla due to decreased ROM of that side. These patients will have difficulty dressing and completing self-care tasks. These patients are also at risk for pressure sores in the arm and hand due to decreased mobility of the affected side. These patients are not at a higher risk for seizures.

137. D: A child who presents with bilateral coordination issues has difficultly using both sides of the body at the same time in a controlled and organized manner. Treatment of these children needs to focus on activities that integrate both sides of the body. Having the child blow bubbles and reach with both hands to pop them is an example of this. Playing with a toy accordion uses both sides as

well. Tearing strips of paper and gluing it on paper also uses the right and left sides of the child's body. Placing the child's hands in sensory buckets does not work on increasing bilateral coordination. This activity would be appropriate for children who are tactile defensive.

138. C: Parkinson disease is a degenerative disease in which both motor and cognition are affected. These patients will benefit from ROM, strength, and coordination activities. This disease is degenerative so energy conservation and retraining for ADLs is also important. Safety issues need to be addressed because memory deficits and dementia can also be present in these patients. Autism is a sensory processing disorder and patients would benefit from sensory integration treatment techniques. CRPS is a chronic pain issue that affects extremities, and carpal tunnel syndrome is median nerve compression in the wrist.

139. D: OT services are appropriate for all age groups regardless of culture and socioeconomic backgrounds. These populations include people with functional impairments, activity limitations, cognitive disabilities, and populations that would benefit from health promotion. OT services are not appropriate to teach people different languages to overcome their language barrier issue.

140. D: OT services are provided at prisons, inpatient/outpatient hospital settings, subacute units, nursing facilities, mental health facilities, inpatient rehabilitation units, and schools. OTs do not provide services at police stations.

141. A: The COTA should be assessing some of the following questions before determining an appropriate treatment activity for the child: Does the child have enough endurance to practice? What is the child's FM like? What is the child's cognitive level? How does the child learn best? Can the child perform symmetrical tasks? Does a verbal explanation help or cause confusion? It is irrelevant how many peers the child gets along with, how many siblings the child has, or if the child is continent.

142. C: A Velcro shoe closure is used with children who are unable to independently tie their shoes. A long-handled shoe horn can be used with children who have decreased ROM and a button hook is used with children who have decreased FM skills. A mouth stick is used for a C1-C3 SCI patient who is unable to use the extremities.

143. A: The COTA is working towards increasing the child's FM skills. Using fastening boards, dressing up dolls, and using a dressing vest that has oversized fasteners to work on FM skills would benefit this child. A dressing stick, long-handled shoe horn, Velcro shoe closure, tumble forms, reacher, zipper grip, sock aid, shoe remover, and button hook are all examples of adaptive equipment. Using these dressing aids will modify the child's environment to make it easier, but will not work on increasing the child's FM skills.

144. A: The child should be placed in a quadruped position to develop the child's trunk and limb co-contraction pattern that is used for crawling. If the therapist places the child in a static standing position, they are working on increasing the strength in the upper body. Prone on elbows is used to inhibit tonic neck reflexes to provide trunk and proximal limb stability and side-lying is used to elicit lateral trunk responses for those dominated by tonic reflexes.

145. D: A TENS unit refers to the use of externally applied electrical stimulation with surface electrodes to decrease a patient's pain. Iontophoresis delivers anti-inflammatory medication transdermally through a patient's skin. A commonly used drug is dexamethasone. Ultrasound can

be used on a pulsed setting, which is commonly used for pain. NMES is used for weak muscles to elicit a stronger muscle contraction for strengthening purposes or gains with ROM.

146. C: A reclining wheelchair is often used with patients after THR. These patients have a hip precaution of no hip flexion past 90. A wheelchair with an adjustable backrest will allow for reclining when the patient is sitting and prevent flexion past 90 degrees of the patient's hip. A low and soft chair is contraindicated for this population because they can be less safe for the patient after THR. A universal cuff is used for people who have UE limitations.

147. B: Rhythmical rotation is used to increase mobility. This technique involves PROM to decrease a patient's spasticity. When a joint is passively stretched slowly, this causes relaxation of the arm and spasticity will decrease, which increases ROM. Active technique and rapid stretch would not be appropriate for a spastic patient and does not refer to rhythmical rotation. Repeated contractions are used by initiating movement and sustaining a contraction through the ROM, which is used to increase both strength and ROM.

148. A: A sequential compression device works to prevent DVTs in a postop THR patient. Inflatable, external leggings provide intermittent pneumatic compression to the legs. A knee immobilizer is used to provide support for the knee when moving in and out of bed and when walking. Balanced suspensions are used to support the affected leg in the first days postop. A reclining wheelchair has an adjustable backrest that is used for patients who have hip flexion precautions.

149. A: Research has shown that the best position for the wrist to decrease intercarpal pressure is having the wrist in neutral and a maximum of 3 degrees in ulnar deviation. Carpal tunnel is when the median nerve is compressed at the wrist in the carpal tunnel. A wrist splint in the proper position will help decrease this pressure and can reduce the symptoms of this diagnosis. All the other options involve splints that place the wrist in a flexed position, which will increase intercarpal pressure and increase the symptoms of this diagnosis.

150. D: A patient who has hypertonia presents with an increase in tone in their arms and leg. This patient would benefit from inhibitory techniques such as slow rocking, neutral warmth, and deep pressure to decrease the patient's tone. A tapping technique is used for patients with hypotonia (decreased tone) and is a facilitatory technique.

151. D: A person diagnosed with Guillain-Barré syndrome often has sensory loss distally along with muscle weakness and stiffness of their extremities. These patients often have pain in their extremities as well due to the increased stiffness associated with this syndrome. Therefore, sensory re-education activities, dynamic splinting, and PREs are appropriate for this patient. A patient with Guillain-Barré syndrome does not have any cognitive deficits, so cognitive perceptual retraining activities are not appropriate.

152. D: A patient who has had a stroke and is in stage 2 of Brunnstrom's stages of motor recovery has active movement that can be facilitated or can occur spontaneously as an associated reaction. Therefore, facilitation of the tonic neck reflex and spinal reflex would initiate active motion. Resistance applied to contralateral side to produce movement is an example of an associated reaction to see movement and is appropriate for a patient at level 2. A patient who has a level 6 has the ability to complete functional tasks and only shows signs of their diagnosis when the nervous system is stressed. Therefore, having the patient complete a timed set of self-care activities would be appropriate.

153. B: The ADA requirements for a house are 32" doorway, 36" hallway, and 31" countertops.

154. A: A person who is in stage 6 of Reisburg's stage of dementia can only complete ADL tasks with cues. They would not be able to complete a complex self-care task without cuing or even a simple self-care or cooking task without cuing.

155. A: The infraspinatus is a prime mover of shoulder external rotation. Therefore, you would not want to initiate ER until the tendon is fully healed and you receive authorization from physician. The subscapularis is the prime mover of IR and the supraspinatus is involved in flexion and abduction of the shoulder.

156. D: The therapist is having the child perform activities that involve coordination of the child's left and right hand. This is working on the skill of bilateral coordination. Sensory processing is not a motor issue. FM and GM strength are not being worked on because the therapist is not having the child do strengthening tasks.

157. A: The main goal is to strengthen the child's hands for increased function for writing tasks. The best activity would be to hide small objects in Theraputty and have the child try to pull out each item. Throwing a ball to the right and left of the child would work on crossing the midline or bilateral coordination. Finger painting activity and shaving cream may be a sensory activity or bilateral coordination but neither is increasing the child's hand strength.

158. D: Osteoarthritis is a degenerative disease of joints often called the "wear and tear" disease of the joints. If the patient presents with both Heberden and Bouchard nodes, the arthritis may be in a more progressive stage. Heat and gentle AROM such as tendon gliding may help to increase the patient's ROM and decrease pain. Often, modifying the environment such as adaptive jar openers or building up handles on utensils can increase the patient's overall function. Aggressive PREs would likely cause a flare-up of arthritis symptoms and would be contraindicated for this patient.

159. C: A C6 level of SCI can perform shoulder flexion, IR, extension, and adduction. They can also do pronation and wrist extension (tenodesis grasp). They will not, however, be able to perform wrist flexion. Wrist flexion is possible with a C7 SCI patient.

160. B: The minimum doorway clearance for wheelchair accessibility is 32". The average wheelchair width is 24-26". 30", 26", and 28" would be too narrow for a wheelchair to fit through the door.

161. C: The National Board for Certification in Occupational Therapy, Inc (NBCOT) does not require a COTA to publish an article to renew their certification. They do require the COTA to complete the entire Certification Renewal Application and abide by the NBCOT Candidate/Certificate Code of Conduct. The COTA is also required to accrue 36 PDU every 3 years in order to renew their NBCOT certification.

162. B: A COTA's main role is the implement of treatment for patients with orders and supervision from an OTR. The COTA is not allowed to evaluate patients. They can only contribute to an evaluation under the supervision of an OTR. The COTA cannot initiate discharge planning unless they have collaborated with the supervising OTR. The COTA's main role is also not to fabricate static and dynamic splints.

163. B: If a person gets their license put on probation, the individual needs to meet a requirement in order to get the license back. Suspension is loss of a license for a specific time. Revocation is permanent loss of a license and ineligibility is the removal of eligibility for a license.

164. A: Revocation of a license is when the license is permanently lost. Loss for a specific time is suspension. Probation is when an individual needs to meet a condition in order to get the license back. Reprimand is a private communication of disapproval of conduct.

165. A: An entry-level COTA needs to be supervised under close supervision by an OTR. They can also be supervised by an advanced COTA under the supervision of an OTR. Routine or general supervision is not allowed for an entry-level COTA. COTAs are allowed to supervise entry-level COTAs as long as they are under the supervision of an OTR.

166. A: Intermediate COTA supervision is routine or general supervision by an OTR or advanced COTA under the supervision of an OTR. This type of COTA does not require close supervision like an entry-level COTA. An advanced COTA requires general supervision by an OTR. COTAs are allowed to be supervised by an advanced COTA under the supervision of an OTR.

167. D: A COTA's main role is to implement treatment with orders from the supervising OTR. They can also have other roles as well. This includes clerical duties, prep area for new treatment session, and CG during transfers. The COTA is not allowed to evaluate the need for OT services. All evaluations must be completed by an OTR. A COTA is allowed to contribute to an evaluation but cannot do it independently.

168. D: Principle 3 is Answer A. Principle 8 is answer B. Principle 4 is answer C. There is no principle in the NBCOT Candidate/Certificant Code of Conduct that states a certificant shall promote the profession of OT by publishing articles to aid in the professional development of the profession.

169. B: The specific purpose of the OT Code of Ethics and Ethic Standards is specifically concerned with the profession of occupational therapy. It is not to provide other domains such as PT and speech therapy standards from which to practice.

170. D: This answer is under principle 2: nonmaleficence. This principle states that OT personnel shall intentionally refrain from actions that cause harm. Therefore, avoiding harm to recipients of OT services fits under this principle.

171. D: The seven core concepts are altruism, equality, freedom, justice, dignity, truth, and prudence.

172. A: The Occupational Safety and Health Administration (OSHA) defines Universal Precautions as an approach to infection control. The concept states that all human blood and certain human bodily fluids are treated if they are known to be infectious for HIV, HBV, and other bloodborne pathogens. Therefore, the first step should be to provide a sterile barrier between you and the patient before any other treatment is initiated.

173. B: An ITP stands for Individual Treatment Plan for a population of birth to 3 years of age. This plan has a focus on family, child, and play. This type of plan is not appropriate for a geriatric population.

174. D: The six types of notes are evaluations, re-evaluations, progress notes, contact notes, transition notes, and discharge notes. A physician's prescription does not fit under this category.

175. B: A student completing a level 1 rotation is gaining experience in various community settings. This not does require an OT practitioner to supervise the student. They can be supervised by non-OT personnel. However, they do need to be supervised.

176. A: The three reimbursable categories for OT are skilled OT services, safety concerns, and prevention of secondary complications. Vocation, leisure, and social issues are not reimbursable service categories. They can be grouped under skilled services depending on the deficit and how it impacts function. Delaying the onset of premorbid symptoms is not a reimbursable service category.

177. D: A therapist must use waterproof black ink when documenting. The therapist must also sign and date every note. A therapist cannot erase mistakes. A therapist can also not use correction fluid to correct the mistake. When a mistake is made, you must draw a line through it and then sign and date the mistake.

178. A: The "O" portion of the note is the health professional's observations. These observations need to be measureable and quantifiable. This does not include the client's or therapist's perception of how the treatment went. The therapist's perception would go under assessment and the client's perception fits under subjective.

179. A: A BIRP note stands for Behavior, Intervention, Response, Plan. The behavior is the therapist's observations and client statements. The intervention is the therapist's methods used to address goals and objectives, observations, and client statements. The response is the client's response to intervention and progress made towards the treatment plan. The plan is the plan for continued treatment based on the client's response.

180. A: MDS stands for Minimum Data Set. It is a note that is used in skilled nursing homes to determine the level of care by assessing all aspects of the patient.

181. B: Eleanor Clarke Slagle. Ruth Brunyate Wiemer was the former AOTA president in 1998. Marion Crampton worked at the Massachusetts Department of Public Health and developed the OTA program in Massachusetts. Mildred Schwagmeyer was assistant director of education at the OTA's national office until 1974.

182. A: Dorothea Dix was a human rights activist who tried to improve public institutions for the mentally ill. Eleanor Clark Slagle was the "mother of OT" who started the first OT school. Marion Crampton worked at the Massachusetts Department of Public Health and developed the OTA program in Massachusetts. Mildred Schwagmeyer was assistant director of education at the OTA's national office until 1974.

183. A: The Procedural Justice principle states that all OT personnel shall comply with institutional rules, local, state, federal, and international laws, and AOTA documents that apply to the OT profession. Principle 3 is Autonomy and Confidentiality and states that OT practitioners have a duty to treat the client according to their desires and to protect their information confidentially. Principle 4 is Social Justice and states that OTs shall provide services in a fair manner. Principle 1 is Beneficence and states that all OT personnel shall demonstrate a concern for the well-being of the recipients of their services.

184. B: Veracity is the principle that states OT personnel shall provide comprehensive, accurate, and objective information when representing the profession. Beneficence states that all OT personnel shall demonstrate a concern for the well-being of the recipients of their services. Fidelity states that OTs shall treat their peers with respect, fairness, and integrity. Procedural Justice states that OTs shall comply with institutional rules, local, state, and federal laws, and AOTA documents that apply to the profession.

185. A: Fidelity states that OT personnel shall treat colleagues and other professionals with respect, fairness, and integrity. Social Justice states that OT personnel shall provide services in a fair and equitable manner. Procedural Justice states that OTs should comply with laws and regulations and AOTA documents that apply to the profession. Veracity is the principle that states OT personnel shall provide accurate and objective information when representing the profession.

186. C: A COTA can perform clerical duties, routine maintenance, and supervise entry-level COTAs while the OTR is away for a few days. They cannot perform evaluations.

187. A: Probation is when a requirement is made for the individual to meet in order to get their license back. Suspension is when the practitioner loses their license for a specific time. Revocation is a permanent loss of license and ineligibility is the removal of eligibility of a membership.

188. A: Ergonomics is the study of a person's movement to complete a task and to modify the environment to prevent injury. Fugue is when a patient takes on the identity of another person. Service competency is a method to make sure that services are provided with a high level of confidence. Assessments are tests given to evaluate a client.

189. C: The physician should already have his own medical history on the patient he is treating. It is more important to focus on the therapy concerns and progress you are seeing in the clinic as a clinician. Objective data should provide ROM measurements that are important for the physician to see. It is also important for the physician to know if the patient is displaying good effort during treatment sessions and is showing up for regularly scheduled appointments.

190. C: A COTA's role is to inform the OTR of any changes that occur with a patient she is treating. After the supervisory OTR has been informed, both the COTA and OTR can collaborate and decide what the next step should be. The COTA cannot independently modify the patient's treatment plan. After the OTR is informed, the COTA can discuss the change with the patient's family or the physician.

191. B: The "S" component of a SOAP note includes what the client reports. This can be limitations, problems, feelings, concerns, goals, and attitudes. The statement that a patient did not show up for his appointment would go under assessment or objective area of the note to indicate what happened during the patient's scheduled treatment time.

192. C: When treating clients in a mental health facility as an OT therapist, you could be working with clients in anger management or stress management groups. This patient population could also benefit from a coping skills group to help them deal with mental health issues. Strength and endurance training is not appropriate for this patient population and would be appropriate for an outpatient hand or rehab setting.

193. A: An OTR/COTA cannot begin to treat any patient with a medical doctor's referral. The therapist cannot do an intake note, progress note, or discharge note before the referral is made. Therefore, the referral needs to be the first step in the intervention process when treating a patient.

194. B: The definition of "nonskilled" therapy is routine or maintenance therapy. "Skilled" therapy refers to therapy that requires decision making and professional education. Safety concerns and nursing home therapy do not define "nonskilled therapy."

195. D: When working in a skilled nursing home, it is important to document function of the patient, any safety concerns for the patient, and a return to home plan for the patient. An ITP is a treatment plan for patients who are birth to 3 years of age with a focus on family, child, and play.

196. D: The COTA's role in treatment for this child can also be to prep the treatment room before the child arrives, with the treatment activities already in place. The COTA can educate the mother on an HEP for home follow-through with activities that will work on FM skills for the child. The COTA is also allowed to schedule follow-up therapy appointments for the child. The COTA is not allowed to initiate discharge planning and discharge the child without collaborating with the supervising OTR.

197. D: Patient confidentially is an important aspect for clinicians. It is important to cover up the patients' names on schedules that are in the open clinic. It is also important not to leave charts on a table with patients' names so that others can see. A clinician cannot discuss a patient's case with others unless it is a treating physician or another medical professional on the patient's case. A clinician who is running late has nothing to do with the concept of client confidentially.

198. A: A reprimand is when a private conversation occurs between the OTR and the COTA in regard to a disapproval of conduct. A loss of license for a certain amount of time is a suspension. A permanent loss of license is a revocation and to contact the AOTA would not qualify under a reprimand.

199. A: An entry-level COTA is allowed to supervise technicians, OT aides, and volunteers. An intermediate COTA can supervise entry-level COTAs and level 1 OT fieldwork students. An advanced-level COTA can supervise an intermediate COTA.

200. C: An intermediate-level COTA is allowed to supervise level 1 OT fieldwork students, entry-level COTAs, and level 1 and level 2 OTA students. They are not allowed to supervise intermediate COTAs, level 2 OT fieldwork students, or advanced level OTs.

Practice Test #2

Practice Questions

1. Which frame of reference is best utilized to increase wrist extension in a patient who is status post-distal radius fracture?
    a. Developmental
    b. Biomechanical
    c. Neurodevelopmental
    d. Sensory Integration

2. Which of the following treatment techniques demonstrates use of the rehabilitative frame of reference?
    a. Teaching a client with a spinal cord injury how to use a universal cuff with a fork for eating
    b. Applying moist heat prior to range of motion exercises for a client with osteoarthritis
    c. Using weight-bearing techniques to decrease tone in the upper extremity of a client who has had a cerebrovascular accident
    d. Teaching a client with chronic pain how to complete progressive relaxation techniques

3. Which of the following tasks can be performed by a COTA once competency has been established?
    a. Determine what evaluation tests and methods are to be used
    b. Develop a treatment plan and goals based on evaluation results
    c. Supervise a newly-hired COTA
    d. Collect data for quarterly screenings in a long-term care facility

4. An elementary school student has been referred for an occupational therapy evaluation due to difficulty with handwriting and fine motor tasks in the classroom. Once the evaluation has been initiated by the OTR, the OTR may assign all of the following tasks to a COTA except:
    a. administer the VMI.
    b. complete a classroom performance checklist with the teacher.
    c. analyze and interpret the scores from the VMI.
    d. score the VMI.

5. When measuring elbow flexion, the axis of the goniometer should be placed on:
    a. the radial tuberosity.
    b. the medial epicondyle of the humerus.
    c. the lateral epicondyle of the humerus.
    d. the head of the radius.

6. A client presents with hypersensitivity of the palmer aspect of the hand following carpal tunnel release surgery. The treatment plan includes a therapist-guided desensitization program. Which stimulus should be introduced first?
    a. Immersing the hand in a bucket of uncooked rice to find hidden objects
    b. Touching the area with cotton balls
    c. Tapping the area with a cotton swab
    d. Applying firm pressure to the area with a piece of velvet

7. A 75-year-old client with Parkinson's disease has had several falls in the past month during activities of daily living. Which statement made by the client indicates a further need for safety education?

    a. "I am able to get into the shower by myself; I hold onto the soap dish handle to help steady myself."

    b. "I take a lot of rest breaks while getting dressed."

    c. "I steady myself at the counter while making a sandwich."

    d. "I have my wife help me get in and out of the car because I am afraid I may fall."

8. Which of the following is not a component of energy conservation?

    a. Take frequent rest breaks

    b. Do as much as you can until you have to rest

    c. Sit versus standing for bathing and dressing tasks

    d. Plan ahead before activities

9. A quadriplegic client complains of dizziness and nausea after being transferred from his bed to his wheelchair. What should be done immediately?

    a. Tilt the locked wheelchair backward so that the client's feet are above his head

    b. Check for a pulse

    c. Call a code blue

    d. Wait for five minutes, as symptoms should diminish after maintaining a seated position

10. Which of the following activities should be used initially with a child who has an inadequate grasp?

    a. Have the child reach for an object and place it in a container

    b. Have the child pick up an item from a table with her arm supported by the table

    c. Place an object into the hand of the child with her arm stabilized on a table

    d. Place an object into the hand of the child who is sitting in a chair with her arm unsupported

11.   A 72-year-old male on your caseload received a total hip arthroplasty two weeks ago. He currently requires maximum assistance for lower body ADLs. He is motivated to meet his goal of performing lower body dressing independently. Which intervention would be most appropriate to initiate immediately?

    a. Perform all dressing from a seated position, bending over to put on clothing up to the knees and then standing with assistance to complete lower body dressing tasks.

    b. Use a dressing stick, sock aid, and long shoehorn to perform lower body dressing tasks.

    c. Use modified techniques such as crossing one leg in order to put on socks and shoes independently

    d. All of the above interventions combined would be most effective

12. What interventions should be used for a client with rheumatoid arthritis who is experiencing an exacerbation in the joints of her hands and feet?
    a. Splinting as needed, strengthening exercises, energy conservation with joint protection education, and adaptive equipment education
    b. Splinting, progressive resistive excises as tolerated, energy conservation with joint protection education, and adaptive equipment education
    c. Splinting as needed, isometric exercises, energy conservation with joint protection education, and adaptive equipment education
    d. Splinting as needed, active and passive range of motion exercises, energy conservation with joint protection education, and adaptive equipment

13. Which of the following is an example of direct occupational therapy services in a school setting?
    a. Observing a student who is not on your caseload in physical education classes
    b. Meeting with a teacher to discuss the implementation of a seat cushion in the classroom
    c. Working on visual perceptual activities with a student who has illegible handwriting
    d. Providing a teacher with a list of pre-writing exercises to use with her kindergarten class

14. Your supervising OTR has asked you to fabricate a resting hand splint for a 35-year-old man who suffered burns to his right hand. What is the purpose of the splint?
    a. To prevent pain
    b. To alleviate pressure on the burned tissues
    c. To allow for optimal blood flow
    d. To prevent deformity of the hand

15. The nursing staff reports that they have noticed reddened skin 30 minutes after removing a client's right hand splint to prevent contractures. What should be done?
    a. Continue with the established schedule for wearing the splint, as redness is to be expected
    b. Decrease the amount of time the client wears the splint by 30 minutes
    c. Discontinue use of the splint until it is re-evaluated and necessary adjustments are made
    d. Discontinue use of the splint, as it is not appropriate

16. A member of the therapy staff is overheard on the elevator telling another staff member that Mr. Jones was just diagnosed with a MRSA infection and to be sure to take precautions. This is an example of what type of violation?
    a. ADA
    b. IDEA
    c. HIPAA
    d. The actions taken were a part of infection control, so no rule has been violated

17. While observing a client in the dining room who has Parkinson's disease, you notice that he is having difficulty with self-feeding due to tremors and dyskinesia. Which piece of adaptive feeding equipment would be most beneficial for this client?
    a. Weighted utensils
    b. Built-up handles on utensils
    c. A universal cuff for utensils
    d. This client would benefit from caregiver assistance for feeding activities

18. While working on grooming techniques for the first time with a client who has had a CVA, you note that she is unable to brush her teeth even though she does not have a sensory, motor, or cognitive deficit that would prevent her from being able to complete this task. This client is most likely exhibiting which one of the following deficits?
    a. Stereoagnosis
    b. Apraxia
    c. Unilateral neglect
    d. Poor visual attention

19. A client with increased tone of the right upper extremity following a CVA would benefit from weight-bearing techniques during seated grooming tasks. What position should the right upper extremity be in for weight-bearing?
    a. Shoulder adducted and internally rotated with the elbow, wrist, and digits in extension
    b. Shoulder adducted and internally rotated with the wrist and digits in extension
    c. Shoulder abducted and externally rotated with the wrist and digits in flexion
    d. Shoulder abducted and externally rotated with the wrist and digits in extension

20. Which of the following adaptive devices would most benefit a client with an SCI who has a lesion at the C6 level?
    a. Universal cuff
    b. Mouth stick
    c. Built up handles
    d. Rocker knife

21. Your client with muscular dystrophy has significant upper extremity muscle weakness. His elbow strength is graded Poor plus (2+) and his shoulder muscular strength ranges from Poor (2) to Fair minus (3-). His endurance for continual activity is poor. Which of the following devices could be used to assist him with upper extremity movements?
    a. Volar cock-up splint
    b. Mobile arm support/balanced forearm orthosis
    c. Suspension sling
    d. Both B and C

22. Accessible rooms are now required in hotels as a result of which Act?
    a. IDEA
    b. ADA
    c. HIPAA
    d. HCFA

23. A type of perceived pain in the amputated limb that often interferes with prosthetic training or prosthetic use is called:
    a. phantom pain.
    b. phantom sensations.
    c. residual limb hyperesthesia.
    d. non-existent pain phenomenon.

24. The client you are working with requires supervision for lower body ADLs. When the patient is performing lower body dressing, what type of support should the therapist provide?
    a. The therapist should have his hands on the patient but not assist with the activity
    b. The therapist should be with the patient while the patient is performing this activity
    c. The therapist should assist with 10-25% of the activity
    d. The therapist should have his hands on the client and assist as needed

25. When beginning stand pivot transfer training with a client who has hemiparesis, which side should the patient lead the transfer with?
    a. The non-involved side
    b. The involved side
    c. The patient can lead with either side
    d. A person with hemiparesis cannot transfer using the stand pivot technique

26 A client who is a 32-year-old male with C7 quadriplegia requires transfer training from bed to wheelchair and wheelchair to bed. He is able to perform scapular depressions and his triceps are intact. What type of transfers would be most beneficial for this client?
    a. Stand pivot
    b. Assisted sliding board transfer
    c. Independent depression transfer
    d. Independent sliding board transfer

27. A 72-year-old female with COPD has been admitted to the sub-acute unit following a three-day stay in an acute care facility. She is unable to complete self-care activities without assistance due to poor endurance and shortness of breath. What should initial treatment sessions focus on?
    a. Energy conservation and work simplification education including breathing techniques
    b. Therapeutic exercises to increase endurance
    c. Homemaking skills
    d. Functional mobility

28. A 75-year-old client is receiving occupational therapy in an acute care facility four days post-op for ORIF of the right femur following a fall at home. Medically, she is stable enough to leave the acute care facility. The client indicated that her discharge plans are to return home to her two-story house where she lives alone. You have noted that she is having difficulty with short-term memory, which affects her ability to safely perform activities of daily living. She is currently performing self-care at a level of minimal-to-moderate assistance. She is able to tolerate 2-3 hours of therapy (total for all therapies) a day. What setting is the most appropriate place to recommend for discharge?
    a. Long-term care facility
    b. Inpatient, rehabilitation facility
    c. Discharge to home with home therapy
    d. Discharge to home with a home health aide 1-2 hours a day

29. A COTA is working with a client with a right hemisphere lesion CVA on grooming tasks. The client is observed to wash the right side of his face and only brushes the right side of his teeth. What type of deficit do these behaviors most likely indicate?
    a. Homonymous hemianopsia
    b. Apraxia
    c. Visual agnosia
    d. Unilateral neglect

30. What is the best way to train a client with low back pain to brush his teeth?
    a. Standing at the sink, only bending over when necessary
    b. Standing with one foot on a stool, bending the knees when needed to rinse
    c. Seated at the sink
    d. Brushing the teeth while standing with both knees bent

31. Which of the following is a compensation for decreased balance?
    a. Spreading the feet apart
    b. Keeping the arms at the sides
    c. Keeping the feet close together
    d. Holding onto objects that are close

32. The evaluation results of a 28-year-old female show numbness in the thumb and the index, middle, and half of the ring fingers; decreased strength in the hand, and a positive Phalen's test. What is most likely causing these symptoms?
    a. Cubital tunnel syndrome
    b. Carpal tunnel syndrome
    c. Epicondylitis
    d. Thoracic outlet syndrome

33. A deformity of the finger with the MPs in extension, the PIP joint in flexion, and the DIP joint in extension is known as:
    a. swan-neck deformity.
    b. mallet finger.
    c. boutonniere deformity.
    d. trigger finger.

34. A 64-year-old female client with multiple sclerosis is wheelchair dependent. She is currently on the OT caseload due to a decline in her ADL functioning. The client has upper extremity weakness and is no longer able to perform weight shifting independently. She is also in need of a new wheelchair cushion. Noting a history of skin integrity issues in her evaluation, which of the following cushions would be the best for this client?
    a. High density foam
    b. Foam cushion with cut-outs at the ischial tuberosities
    c. Foam cushion with sheepskin covering
    d. Gel cushion

35. Which of the following therapeutic modalities is contraindicated for a client with RSD of the upper extremity?
    a. Relaxation training
    b. Passive stretching
    c. Paraffin
    d. Stress loading

36. A client has been having difficulties with handwriting tasks in the classroom. The teacher reports that the client is unable to keep up with the class when taking notes and it has had an effect on his grades. The client has been complaining of fatigue with longer handwriting tasks. Upon observation, you note that the student holds his pencil with a quadruped grasp in neutral. He appears labored while writing and uses heavy pressure on his writing implement. What modifications would best address this client's needs in the classroom?

    a. The use of a keyboard for writing tasks

    b. A slanted surface for writing and a pencil grip to promote dynamic tripod grasp

    c. A slanted surface for writing, a mechanical pencil, and a teacher-provided outline to decrease demands

    d. A seat for the client close to the front of the room and a pencil grip

37. A teacher reports that her student who has been diagnosed with autism has been covering his ears and screaming when there is a loud, unexpected sound. She also reports that he is unable to attend to tasks when there are distracting noises in the background, such as the air conditioner running or other kids playing outside at recess. Which of the following interventions would most likely help this student?

    a. Noise-blocking headphones

    b. Desensitization to loud noises

    c. Removing the child from the room when there is too much noise

    d. Moving the student to a different class with less noise

38. Which of the following could be used to inhibit spasticity?

    a. Tapping the muscle belly

    b. Using vibration over the muscle belly

    c. Icing

    d. Slow rocking

39. Which of the following can elicit lip closure when working on feeding with a child?

    a. Pushing up on the lower jaw

    b. Brushing the lips

    c. Using verbal commands to close the lips

    d. Applying deep pressure to both cheeks

40. The supervising occupational therapist has requested that the COTA administer two subsections of the Bruininks-Oseretsky Motor Development Scale. The COTA has never administered this standardized test before. What should the COTA do?

    a. Administer the test since it is standardized and the instructions are self-explanatory

    b. Review the test manual prior to testing

    c. Explain to the OTR that she is not competent in administering that particular test and therefore cannot administer it

    d. Refuse to administer the test as COTAs are not qualified to administer standardized tests.

41. In working with a client who has a generalized response following a head injury, which of the following techniques of sensory stimulation should not be used?

    a. Soft textures to provide tactile input

    b. A pinprick to elicit a pain response

    c. A family member addressing the client by name

    d. Familiar smells

42. Which of the following sensory systems is responsible for telling us where our bodies are in space?
    a. Vestibular
    b. Tactile
    c. Visual
    d. Proprioceptive

43. Where should the axis of the goniometer be placed when measuring wrist extension?
    a. The styloid process of the radius
    b. The CMC joint of the first digit
    c. The dorsal aspect of the wrist joint in between the radius and the ulna
    d. The ulnar styloid

44. Placing a client on a platform swing for a ball activity will provide increased input to which sensory system?
    a. Olfactory
    b. Proprioceptive
    c. Tactile
    d. Vestibular

45. When placed a in supine position and the head is turned to one side, the limbs on one side of the body will have increased extensor tone and those on the other side have increased flexor tone. Which brain stem reflex has been elicited?
    a. Symmetrical tonic neck reflex (STNR)
    b. Asymmetrical tonic neck reflex (ATNR)
    c. Tonic labyrinthine reflex (TLR)
    d. Associated reaction

46. Which of the following is not a symptom of reflex sympathetic dystrophy (RSD) of the hand?
    a. Edema
    b. Color changes in the skin
    c. Absence of sensation
    d. Excessive sweating

47. Which of the following activities would be best to help increase postural strength of a 6-year-old child with flaccid cerebral palsy?
    a. Laying supine to watch a movie
    b. Standing in a standing frame to complete a puzzle
    c. Working on a puzzle in the prone position
    d. Working on a puzzle while seated at a table

48. While working with a client who is two-weeks post CVA, she complains of pain in her left lower extremity. She cries out in pain when you touch her left calf and reports pain when you passively move her foot into dorsiflexion. You also note edema in the extremity. What should you do?
    a. Call 911
    b. Report the findings to a nurse or physician
    c. Try to have client work through the pain
    d. Report the findings to her physical therapist when you get a chance

49. Which of the following activities would be the most difficult while weight bearing on an upper extremity with spasticity?
    a. Standing at a counter to put groceries away in an overhead cabinet
    b. Using both upper extremities to wipe down a table
    c. Wiping down a mat with an uninvolved extremity while in the quadruped position
    d. Reaching for cones with an uninvolved extremity while weight shifting and seated on a mat table

50. Which of the following is the best way to modify an activity to increase a balance challenge when working with a client who has decreased sitting balance?
    a. Incorporating reach into the activity
    b. Adding weights to the activity
    c. Making objects smaller
    d. Providing a stable surface to work on

51. A 75-year-old woman reports difficulty with upper extremity dressing due to decreased ROM. She has decreased internal rotation and flexion of the shoulders bilaterally. Which of the following adaptive techniques would most benefit her?
    a. Using a front-closure bra and compensatory dressing techniques
    b. Using a button hook
    c. Using adaptive clothing
    d. Using a back-closure bra and compensatory dressing techniques

52. A three-in-one commode can be used for all the following except as a:
    a. bedside commode.
    b. raised seat over the commode.
    c. chair for tub transfer.
    d. shower chair.

53. Which of the following activities would be the best to use with a 78-year-old female client to work on standing balance and endurance?
    a. Playing an XBOX game while standing
    b. Coloring a picture on an incline board while standing at a table
    c. Playing solitaire while standing
    d. Standing to put nuts on bolts that are secured to the wall

54. When positioning a hemiplegic patient supine in bed, support should be as follows:
    a. A pillow should be placed under the affected shoulder and under the affected hip
    b. A pillow should be placed under the feet to prevent edema in the lower extremities
    c. A pillow should be placed under the unaffected shoulder and under the unaffected hip
    d. A pillow should be placed under the low back and under the knees

55. Which of the following could be used to improve triceps that are rated Poor minus?
    a. Lying supine to perform triceps extensions with 1-lb. weights
    b. Using a Thera-Band for resistance to extend the elbow while standing or in a seated position
    c. Wearing an arm skate to perform flexion and extension while seated at a table or lying supine on a mat table
    d. Performing active triceps extensions against gravity

56. When a client is exercising, what is expected to happen to the blood pressure?
    a. Systolic will go up, diastolic will go down
    b. Systolic will go up and diastolic will stay the same
    c. Both systolic and diastolic will increase
    d. Blood pressure is unchanged by exercise

57. When measuring the armrest height of a wheelchair, how many inches should be added to the seat- to-elbow (flexed at 90 degrees) measurement?
    a. ½ inch
    b. ¾ inch
    c. 1 inch
    d. 2 inches

58. Which activity is most appropriate for a client who is three weeks' post-myocardial infarction?
    a. Walking up and down stadium stairs
    b. Walking for 20 minutes on a treadmill
    c. Spending 30 minutes in a sauna
    d. Shoveling snow off the driveway

59. A 10-year-old client has been having difficulty in gym class and has been bumping into others with force while trying to participate in organized ball games. Which of the following activities would be best for working on body awareness?
    a. Obstacle courses that require several different types of movement (jumping, crashing, hopping, etc.)
    b. Swinging
    c. Working on table-top activities that are calming prior to gym class
    d. A behavior plan with positive reinforcement for not bumping into others

60. A new client has been placed on the occupational therapy caseload following admission to a long-term care setting. The OT evaluation indicates that the client has been agitated and has been refusing care from staff. The client is not oriented to place and has decreased short-term memory. Initial OT treatment that would best benefit this client would be to:
    a. place physical reminders in the client's room for orientation, establish routines, and educate staff to initiate care by verbally explaining to the client where he is and what they are doing.
    b. begin exercises to improve short-term memory, such as games of concentration and cards.
    c. use repetition to improve the client's memory and to help him become oriented to place.
    d. provide calendars and alarms as reminders.

61. Which of the following devices may be used to help a client who has demonstrated difficulty staying seated in her desk at school due to sensory issues?
    a. Weighted blanket
    b. Weighted lap pad
    c. Fidget toy
    d. Chewy toy for times when seated at her desk

62. A client who is described as sensory avoiding:
    a. has low sensory registration.
    b. is often unaware of touch.
    c. is often impulsive.
    d. is often described as defensive.

63. How long should hip precautions be followed after a total hip replacement?
    a. One week
    b. Three weeks
    c. Six months
    d. As determined by the surgeon

64. A person with left brain damage can have deficits in what area?
    a. Long-term memory
    b. Language
    c. Perception
    d. Short-term memory

65. Which of the following can help decrease the pain of an acute case of lateral epicondylitis?
    a. Moist heat
    b. Ice massage
    c. Resistive exercise
    d. None of these

66. When performing a dependent stand pivot transfer, the caregiver should block the client's:
    a. feet.
    b. hips.
    c. knees.
    d. chest.

67. The OT has asked a COTA to work with a client on ADLs. The COTA reviews the chart and notes that the client requires maximum assistance for ADLs and functional transfers. Upon entering the room, the COTA notes that the client is rather large and she is unsure if she can perform the bed-to-wheelchair transfer alone. What should she do?
    a. Leave the client in bed
    b. Attempt the transfer by herself
    c. Ask someone to assist her with the transfer
    d. Attempt the transfer and stop to get help if she cannot complete it

68. When should universal precautions be used?
    a. When the client's family is present
    b. When regulatory inspections are done
    c. When coming in contact with body fluids
    d. When the therapist feels it may be necessary

69. Which of the following are components of Brunnstrum's flexor synergy of the upper extremity?
    a. External rotation of the shoulder, elbow flexion, and forearm pronation
    b. Internal rotation of the shoulder, elbow flexion, and forearm supination
    c. External rotation of the shoulder, elbow extension, and forearm supination
    d. External rotation of the shoulder, elbow flexion, and forearm supination

70. What time of day is it best for a client to wear a static splint that has been designed to prevent contractures?
   a. First thing in the morning
   b. All day
   c. In the evening
   d. While sleeping

71. What PNF pattern is used when brushing hair on the side opposite that which the client is holding the brush?
   a. D1 flexion
   b. D1 extension
   c. D2 flexion
   d. D2 extension

72. What method should be used for wrapping a residual limb after amputation?
   a. Wrap proximal to distal in a circular method, overlapping by ¼ the width of the bandage
   b. Wrap distal to proximal in a circular method, overlapping ¼ the width of the bandage
   c. Wrap distal to proximal using a figure-eight method
   d. Wrap proximal to distal using a figure-eight method

73. When working with a client who has an above-the-knee amputation, ADL training should be done:
   a. with the prosthesis on.
   b. without the prosthesis.
   c. both with and without the prosthesis.
   d. whatever way the client indicates he will do activities at home.

74. The teacher of a student who is on consultative OT services reports that the student has been hitting other kids and being disruptive during circle time. The client is on services due to sensory issues, one being tactile defensiveness. While observing circle time, you note that children are seated very close together and often touching one another. What recommendations would be best for this client?
   a. Ask the teacher to use carpet squares during circle time
   b. Keep the student seated at his chair during circle time
   c. Reward the student with a sticker chart for sitting in circle time without disruption
   d. Have students leave extra space around the client

75. Which of the following tasks is considered an IADL?
   a. Meal preparation
   b. Opening a door
   c. Shaving
   d. Brushing the teeth

76. Working on copying 3D block designs can help improve what type of apraxia?
   a. Ideational
   b. Ideomotor
   c. Dressing
   d. Constructional

77. What treatment method would work best for a client who is post-CVA and who requires maximum assistance to wash his face due to ideational apraxia?
    a. Give the client verbal instructions while he performs the task
    b. Teach the task one step at a time using tactile and verbal instructions
    c. Demonstrate the task before asking him to do it
    d. Perform the entire task hand over hand and then have him complete the task

78. Shaping and reinforcement are examples of what approach to treatment?
    a. Sensory integration
    b. Adaptive
    c. Applied behavior analysis
    d. Cognitive

79. Which type of muscle contraction does not involve the movement of a joint?
    a. Isotonic
    b. Concentric
    c. Eccentric
    d. Isometric

80. Which of the following is a contraindication for paraffin?
    a. Status post-fracture
    b. Open wound
    c. Decreased ROM
    d. Pain

81. When performing passive range of motion on a client with quadriplegia, what position should the wrist be in while flexing the fingers?
    a. Flexion
    b. Neutral
    c. Extension
    d. It does not matter

82. How wide must a doorway be to accommodate a wheelchair?
    a. 20 inches
    b. 26 inches
    c. 30 inches
    d. 32 inches

83. When a client who is in a coma following a brain injury is quickly moved from side-lying to a supine position, the following motor response is noted: shoulder adduction, flexion and internal rotation, elbow flexion, forearm pronation and wrist and fingers flexed on the chest. His lower extremities are in extension, with adduction and internal rotation. This motor response is known as:
    a. Rancho's withdrawal response.
    b. decerebrate rigidity.
    c. decorticate rigidity.
    d. a specific response.

84. Which of the following is a principle of joint protection?
    a. Plan ahead
    b. Take frequent rest breaks
    c. Hold positions as long as possible
    d. Stop an activity if it is painful

85. Using your forearms and shoulders to carry an object versus your hands is a principle of what type of education?
    a. Joint protection
    b. Energy conservation
    c. Work simplification
    d. Home safety

86. Multiple sclerosis symptoms can be exacerbated by which of the following?
    a. Exercise
    b. Hot temperatures
    c. Time of day
    d. Atmospheric pressure

87. Ulnar drift is a deformity associated with which diagnosis?
    a. Multiple sclerosis
    b. Rheumatoid arthritis
    c. Amyotrophic lateral sclerosis
    d. Lupus

88. The ability to take in sensory input and regulate an appropriate response is known as:
    a. behavior.
    b. modulation.
    c. response output.
    d. execution.

89. Which of the following supports can be used to help a client who is leaning to the side in a standard wheelchair?
    a. Abduction wedge
    b. Lateral supports
    c. Firm seat insert
    d. Detachable armrest

90. When writing a SOAP note, which of the following statements would be used for the "S" portion of the note?
    a. The patient is able to complete lower body dressing with minimal assistance using assistive devices with verbal cues for safety.
    b. The patient will continue to work on functional balance and safety awareness to achieve a level of modified independence for lower body dressing.
    c. The patient reports that he feels more stable when putting on his pants.
    d. The patient worked on ADL retraining, standing endurance, and functional standing balance activities.

91. A home program for splinting to prevent contractures for a client with rheumatoid arthritis should include which of the following?
   a. A splint-wearing schedule
   b. Instructions on splint modification at home
   c. A description of the type of splint material used
   d. The pattern used for splint fabrication

92. The OTR has asked the COTA to work with a 54-year-old client who has recently suffered bilateral total vision loss following a trauma. While working with the client in the dining room what method would be best for finding food on a plate when a caregiver is present?
   a. Feel for food textures
   b. Have the caregiver feed the client
   c. Use the clock method to describe to the client where the food is
   d. Have the client locate the food independently and then tell the client what the food item is

93. In reviewing the evaluation of a client with a traumatic brain injury, you note that the client is at a level V in the Rancho Los Amigos Scale. Which of the following activities would be best for a client at this level?
   a. Meal preparation tasks
   b. Wiping the face when handed a washcloth
   c. Independent self-feeding
   d. Performing a new task once it has been demonstrated

94. Which activity would be appropriate for a client who is at Level III (localized response) on the Rancho Los Amigos scale?
   a. Matching simple pictures
   b. Completing a ten-piece puzzle
   c. Finishing simple crossword puzzles
   d. Copying 3D block designs

95. How does an occupational therapy assistant get a license to practice?
   a. Applying for each state of practice through the AOTA
   b. Applying to an individual state agency
   c. Applying for each state of practice through the NBCOT
   d. Once an assistant receives a passing score on the certification exam, licensure is automatic

96. Which of the following environmental factors can contribute to falls?
   a. Room temperature
   b. Low lighting
   c. Poor posture
   d. Ear infections

97. In working on self-feeding tasks with a client who is bedridden due to advanced MS, what position should the client be in for safe and effective swallowing?

    a. Upright with the hips at or near a 90-degree angle, maintaining the position for 10-20 minutes after the meal

    b. Upright with the hips at or near a 45-degree angle, maintaining the position for 10-20 minutes after the meal

    c. The head propped with 3-4 pillows, maintaining an upright position for 10-20 minutes after the meal

    d. Upright with the hips at or near a 90-degree angle throughout the meal and maintaining the position for 5 minutes after the meal

98. While working on self-feeding with an 80-year-old client, you note that he is spilling liquids and having difficulty drinking from a cup due to range limitations in shoulder flexion. Which of the following adaptive devices may help this client?

    a. Weighted cup

    b. T-shaped handled mug for drinking

    c. Larger (higher) cup

    d. Nosey (nose cut-out) cup

99. Which of the following tasks can be performed by an occupational therapy aide?

    a. Work on a dynamic standing activity with a client, grading activity as needed

    b. Work on lower body dressing with a client, utilizing adaptive equipment when the aide feels it is necessary

    c. Prepare and apply hot packs to a client under the direct supervision of a therapist or therapy assistant after competency has been established

    d. Supervise and educate a client as needed while performing meal preparation assigned by the COTA as a part of OT treatment

100. A 75-year-old client with Alzheimer's has been referred to occupational therapy after falling from her wheelchair. In reviewing the occupational therapy evaluation, you note that the client fell forward out of her chair while attempting to stand, resulting in a laceration to her head. The client has poor standing balance and reportedly is able to stand halfway up for 2-3 seconds before falling. The client becomes disoriented at times and has significant memory deficits. She is currently in a standard wheelchair with a foam pad. Which of the following initial interventions would be best to try for this client?

    a. A seatbelt to keep her in her seat

    b. A wedge cushion to help keep her seated

    c. A full lap tray

    d. Anti-tipping devices

101. Which of the following is an example of indirect supervision of a COTA by an OTR?

    a. Observation

    b. Email discussions

    c. Co-treatment

    d. Weekly meetings

102. A 9-year-old client who has decreased perceptual skills (especially in the areas of figure-ground and spatial relations) is having a difficult time finding books and folders that he needs in the classroom. Which of the following interventions would be most beneficial for this student?
    a. Put books in different areas of the room
    b. Use a color-coded filing system in his desk
    c. Utilize preferential seating in the front of the room
    d. Use a weighted lap pad to provide input and to increase organization

103. Which of the following activities would be best to work on bilateral integration with a 10-year-old girl who has a diagnosis of Asperger's?
    a. Pinching Theraputty
    b. Playing UNO and card games
    c. Painting a picture frame
    d. Ripping paper for a decoupage craft activity

104. A client with COPD in a sub-acute unit improved her ADL status from maximum assistance at admission to her current level of minimum assistance and supervision for self-care. Her prior level of function was modified independent/supervised for self-care ADLs. The client has not made significant improvement over the past 10 days and the COTA feels that she has met her maximum potential. The physical limitations of the COPD are keeping her from meeting her long-term goal of supervision for all ADLs. The COTA who is treating this client feels that she is ready for discharge from services. Which of the following steps should the COTA take?
    a. Inform social services and discharge the client from OT services
    b. Review the client's status with the OTR and collaborate with the OTR for discharge from services
    c. Continue to treat the client until the OTR decides to discharge the client
    d. Continue to work with the client until the prior level of function is achieved

105. What is the name of the statement by the AOTA that upholds and maintains the standards of conduct within the profession of occupational therapy?
    a. Code of Ethics
    b. Professional Conduct Standards
    c. Practice Act
    d. Professional Practice standards

106. A post-CVA client who exhibits uncontrollable laughing or crying which seems disproportionate to the situation is most likely experiencing which of the following?
    a. Emotional lability
    b. Perseveration
    c. Depression
    d. Decreased frustration tolerance

107. Which of the following leisure activities would be best for a client with a spinal cord injury at the C8/T1 level who was physically active as a runner and a soccer player prior to his injury?
    a. Card games
    b. Billiards
    c. Wheelchair basketball
    d. Board games

108. At what level of spinal cord injury is it first possible to drive a car with hand controls?
   a. C5
   b. C6
   c. C7
   d. C8/T1

109. Which of the following is not used as method of stress management?
   a. Progressive relaxation techniques
   b. Self-assessment techniques
   c. Breathing techniques
   d. Time management techniques

110. Businesses with more than 15 workers, regardless of their source of funding, are required to make provisions for those with disabilities as a part of which legislation?
   a. Rehabilitation Act
   b. Social Security Act
   c. Americans with Disabilities Act
   d. Architectural Barriers Act

111. A client who works in a factory caught his arm in a machine resulting in a crush injury. His occupational therapy evaluation indicates decreased functional use of his right upper extremity secondary to edema, as well as decreased range of motion and decreased strength. The treatment plan includes the following modalities: edema control, ROM/therapeutic exercises, functional activities, and client education. Which of the following activities would be best to use first with this client?
   a. Retrograde massage followed by active range of motion
   b. Retrograde massage followed by pulley exercises
   c. Retrograde massage followed by passive range of motion
   d. Functional activities such as sanding or using nuts and bolts

112. What is the name of the device used by people with physical limitations to operate electronic or computer-based equipment by remote control?
   a. EDU
   b. ECD
   c. CUE
   d. ECU

113. Who is responsible for making legislative and policy decisions in the AOTA?
   a. The Representative Assembly
   b. The Executive Board
   c. The Commission on Ethics
   d. The Commission on Practice

114. In treating a client with osteogenesis imperfecta, what precautions should be taken?
   a. Do not overexert the muscles, as fatigue is an issue.
   b. Be aware of seizure precautions: no flashing lights, control any vestibular input.
   c. There is a high potential to develop contractures. Stretching and splinting needs must be addressed.
   d. There is a high risk of fractures, so the treatment approach must be gentle.

115. A COTA is reviewing an evaluation of a 16-month-old client with a diagnosis of developmental delay who has been referred for early intervention services. She notes that he is able to roll over independently, and sit with support, but is unable to sit independently. At what age does a typical child sit independently?
    a. 6 months
    b. 9 months
    c. 12 months
    d. 14 months

116. Which of the following activities would be best to work on tip pinch with a 3-year-old child who has decreased fine motor control?
    a. Making a picture with Cheerios
    b. Building a block tower
    c. Finger painting
    d. Ripping paper into small pieces

117. While working with an eight-year-old child with cerebral palsy on self-feeding, you note that he has adequate elbow flexion for hand-to-mouth movements but he has limited wrist and finger motion. What piece of adaptive equipment would you try first?
    a. Spoon with a built-up handle
    b. Rocker knife
    c. Curved spoon with a built-up handle
    d. Spork

118. What are the programs to prevent cumulative trauma injuries in the workplace called?
    a. Injury prevention programs
    b. Ergonomic programs
    c. Employee assistance programs
    d. Worksite analysis programs

119. Which of the following is not a cause of cumulative trauma injuries?
    a. The amount of force required for a job
    b. The postures sustained and the positions required
    c. Repetitive motions
    d. Shift work

120. In reviewing the occupational therapy evaluation of a client with cerebral palsy, the COTA notes the following: fluctuations in tone in all extremities, no limitations in ROM, protective reactions are present; and the client has writhing, involuntary movements noted at rest and during purposeful movements. What classification of cerebral palsy would these symptoms indicate?
    a. Flaccid
    b. Spastic
    c. Athetoid
    d. Ataxic

121. Educating a client on how to perform self-inspections after a spinal cord injury is vital to prevent all of the following except:
    a. contractures.
    b. decubitus ulcers.
    c. bruising.
    d. fungal infections.

122. All of the following can contribute to skin breakdown except:
    a. cold.
    b. heat.
    c. shearing.
    d. prolonged positioning.

123. Following trauma, injury, or surgery, a bone can develop in an abnormal location with symptoms of warmth, redness, swelling, and a decrease in range of motion. This is known as:
    a. osteotropic calcification.
    b. orthostatic increase.
    c. heterotopic ossification.
    d. osteoporosis disuse syndrome.

124. Copper tooling on a template is an activity to use with clients in a mental health setting because:
    a. it does not require decision-making.
    b. it helps strengthen finger flexors.
    c. successful outcomes can increase self-esteem.
    d. there are no guidelines or limits.

125. In order to decrease pressure on the median nerve at the carpal ligament, the wrist should be positioned:
    a. in neutral alignment.
    b. in 15-30 degrees of flexion.
    c. in 15-30 degrees of extension.
    d. in 15 degrees of ulnar deviation.

126. Which of the following activities is best used to work on stereognosis?
    a. Submerging the hand in rice to collect small balls
    b. Touching different materials with the vision occluded and then identifying soft vs. hard items
    c. Identifying places on the arm that have been touched with a cotton ball
    d. Reaching for coins in a purse and identifying them

127. A client who has had a total hip arthroplasty will return to his apartment where there is only a tub shower. The client's previous level of function was independent but he has a history of falls. He is currently at a level of supervision, but is expected to reach a level of modified independence when he is discharged. What type of adaptive equipment would you recommend the client use for bathing?
    a. The client should perform sponge baths
    b. A shower chair, grab bars, long-handled sponge, and a long shower hose
    c. A tub transfer bench, long-handled sponge, and long shower hose
    d. Three-in-one commode and long shower hose

128. Which of the following activities places the greatest force on the spine?
    a. Bending at the waist to pick up a piece of paper off of the ground
    b. Swaying from side to side
    c. Turning to reach for something to the side
    d. Reaching overhead

129. The use of group therapy sessions can be effective for individuals with traumatic brain injuries because:
    a. they provide structured social interactions.
    b. they focus on individual goals.
    c. they allow clients to interact with others in an unstructured environment.
    d. they provide additional treatment outside of individual sessions.

130. A prosthetic sock is:
    a. worn over the prosthesis to protect it.
    b. worn under the prosthesis to protect the skin.
    c. worn when the prosthesis is not on to protect the skin and stump.
    d. used to store the prosthesis when it is not being used.

131. A COTA who is competent in the use of a volumeter is taking measurements to see what effect a treatment has on a client with a crush injury. A volumeter is used to measure:
    a. finger edema.
    b. hand edema.
    c. finger circumference.
    d. force of grip.

132. Which of the following activities is best used to work on figure-ground discrimination with a 9-year-old student who has ADHD?
    a. Stringing various colored beads
    b. Cutting curved lines
    c. Copying simple and three-dimensional block designs
    d. Retrieving all of the blue chips from a box of various colored chips

133. Teaching a client with short-term memory impairment due to early stage dementia to repeat his room number in order to find his room is called:
    a. repetition.
    b. chunking.
    c. rehearsal.
    d. recall.

134. What angle should a wheelchair be placed in relation to the surface the client is transferring to for most transfers?
    a. 30 degrees
    b. 45 degrees
    c. 90 degrees
    d 180 degrees

135. Which of the following would benefit an 80-year-old woman who has a diagnosis of COPD to practice meal preparation activities upon return to home?
   a. Place food, cooking utensils, and serving items used the most at counter level
   b. Use built-up handles on cooking utensils
   c. Use a rocker knife for cutting vegetables
   d. Place non-slip mats under mixing bowls

136. Which of the following tactile input would be best to initially advise a parent to provide to a 6-year-old boy with Asperger's who has tactile defensiveness?
   a. Deep pressure input
   b. Light pressure input
   c. Both deep and light pressure input
   d. Advise the parent to avoid touch whenever possible

137. Which of the following would be most beneficial for home management tasks to a 47-year-old female with rheumatoid arthritis?
   a. Move all dishes to counter height
   b. Use extended handles on brooms, dustpans, and mops
   c. Pull out shelves in the kitchen
   d. Use a jar opener

138. An 18-month-old girl who suffered a CVA in utero has left hemiparesis and typically does not use her left hand for any activities. What activity would be best to incorporate bilateral upper extremity use?
   a. Stringing small beads
   b. Copying block designs
   c. Finger painting
   d. Taking apart pop beads

139. When working with a group of 9-year-old boys in fine motor tasks, the COTA notes that they are having difficulty following directions and attending to the work. The COTA institutes a behavior modification system where the boys earn chips for following directions and completing tasks. Chips can be traded in for prizes at the end of the session. What type of behavior modification system is this an example of?
   a. Positive reinforcement
   b. Negative reinforcement
   c. Punishment
   d. Earned behavior

140. While working on self-feeding with a 23-year-old client who has had a traumatic brain injury, the COTA notes that he is coughing and his voice changes when he is drinking. The COTA does not have competency in swallowing skills, as speech therapy addresses swallowing issues in the facility. The COTA has limited experience when she assisted the speech therapist on a couple of occasions. What should the COTA do?
   a. Discuss the symptoms with the OTR and make a referral for speech therapy
   b. Ask the client to tuck his chin when he swallows, as that is what the SLP does
   c. Continue working with the client, as these symptoms are typical following a TBI
   d. Add some thickener to his beverages

141. Why must occupational therapy assistants complete professional development and/or continuing education units?
    a. To renew certification through the NBCOT, as well as to maintain state licensure.
    b. To renew state licensure only.
    c. To renew certification through the NBCOT and state licensing, depending on the states in which it is required.
    d. Continuing education is not required for occupational therapy assistants.

142. The supervision requirements for occupational therapy assistants are regulated by:
    a. the NBCOT.
    b. state regulatory bodies.
    c. individual employers.
    d. the occupational therapist who provides supervision for the assistant.

143. The COTA is examining a switch on a battery-operated toy for a 12-year-old with severe spasticity and very limited motor control. What type of switch would be most beneficial to meet the needs of this client?
    a. Joystick
    b. Standard keyboard
    c. Single switch
    d. Expanded keyboard

144. Which of the following is not a professional development unit (PDU) as defined by the NBCOT?
    a. Performing a self-assessment
    b. Attending AOTA-approved workshops
    c. Developing a professional development plan
    d. Attending a new staff orientation class

145. Which of the following statements is true?
    a. All states have the same continuing competency requirements for certified occupational therapy assistants.
    b. NBCOT regulations differ depending on the jurisdiction of practice.
    c. NBCOT is a national certification that complements state requirements.
    d. Some states do not require certification by the NBCOT.

146. The caregiver of a 76-year-old client with Parkinson's confides to the treating COTA that she is fearful that she will be unable to care for her spouse upon his discharge from the rehabilitation facility. What should the COTA do in this situation?
    a. Reassure her that she will be fine and continue to provide caregiver education
    b. Recommend that she place her spouse in long-term care
    c. Contact the social worker for her to discuss her concerns about discharge and continue to provide caregiver education
    d. Tell the caregiver to hire someone to help at home

147. Which of the following is a performance area as defined by Uniform Terminology for Occupational Therapy?
    a. Cognitive components
    b. Play
    c. Social aspects
    d. Perceptual processing

148. Taking into account a client's cultural beliefs is a part of what domain of uniform terminology?
    a. Performance contexts
    b. Performance components
    c. Performance areas
    d. Performance adjustments

149. The occupational therapist in an acute care center has asked a COTA to treat a client with a flexor tendon repair following the initial evaluation. The COTA has never treated a client with this diagnosis and is uncomfortable with administering the treatment. How should the COTA respond?
    a. The COTA should explain to the OTR that he is unable to administer occupational therapy treatments to this client, as he does not have the competence to treat this diagnosis.
    b. The COTA should educate himself on treatment of this diagnosis and work with the client.
    c. The COTA should apply general knowledge to treat this client, as he is licensed and should be able to treat any diagnosis.
    d. The COTA should report to the rehabilitation department director that he refuses to treat the client.

150. A COTA with ten years of experience can supervise which of the following?
    a. Entry level OTRs, COTAs, and OT aides
    b. Entry level COTAs and OT aides
    c. OT aides
    d. COTAs do not perform supervisory duties

151. Evidenced-based practice is the best approach for a client based on:
    a. research evidence, knowledge, and clinical judgment.
    b. research evidence alone.
    c. clinical judgments alone.
    d. the technique that worked with a previous client with the same diagnosis.

152. Which of the following is considered durable medical equipment that is covered by Medicare?
    a. Reacher
    b. Wheelchair
    c. Transfer tub bench
    d. Elastic shoelaces

153. A client asks the COTA that is treating him to go to dinner after his therapy session. The COTA is attracted to the client and decides that it is fine as long as they don't tell anyone. The COTA and the client develop a sexual relationship outside of the clinic and begin to see each other outside of their scheduled treatment times. Which of the following statements is true regarding this relationship?
    a. The relationship is fine as long as the COTA's supervisors do not find out about it.
    b. The COTA has violated a principal of the Code of Ethics and Standards.
    c. As long as the COTA maintains a professional relationship in the clinic with the client, it does not matter what she does on her personal time.
    d. The COTA should report the relationship to her supervisors to get approval.

154. What is the best response when working with a delusional client who reports that all of the staff are trying to hurt him?
    a. "No one here is trying to hurt you; it's all in your head."
    b. "That must make you feel nervous."
    c. "I'll make sure no one hurts you, so you don't need to worry."
    d. "I wonder why they would try to hurt you?"

155. Which of the following would be best to include in the education of a caregiver who is caring for a client with Alzheimer's?
    a. The importance of taking the client out into the community
    b. Establishing routines for daily activities
    c. How to perform daily range of motion exercises
    d. How to quiz the client to test his memory

156. A 75-year-old is receiving occupational therapy in an acute care setting following a transient ischemic attack; he is at a level of modified independence for self-care as he continues to demonstrate decreased coordination in his right upper extremity. He requires supervision for home management tasks due to mild cognitive deficits. He will be discharged from the acute care hospital in one to two days when he is medically stable. Which setting would be the most appropriate for this client after he is discharged?
    a. Discharge to home with a spouse who is retired and who can supervise or assist with ADLs, as well as referral for outpatient occupational therapy
    b. Discharge to long-term care with referral for occupational therapy
    c. Discharge to a rehabilitation or sub-acute setting
    d. Discharge to home with a spouse and a daily home health aide, plus home occupational therapy

157. Which of the following is an example of a long-term goal?
    a. The client will put on and take off his shoes independently in 2 out of 5 trials
    b. The client will increase standing balance to F+ in order to put on and take of his pants with minimal assistance 75% of the time
    c. The client will perform lower body dressing independently
    d. The client will perform lower body dressing with minimal assistance in 3 out of 5 trials with verbal cues for safety

158. When writing progress notes, which of the following should be included?
    a. Referral source
    b. Client problem list
    c. Prior level of function
    d. Client response to treatment

159. Which of the following statements is true regarding a problem oriented medical record (POMR)?
    a. The POMR has separate sections for each discipline.
    b. The POMR is only used for initial evaluations.
    c. The POMR includes an interdisciplinary plan of treatment based on a list of client problems.
    d. The POMR does not contain subjective data.

160. Which of the following adaptive techniques would be best to help a client who has difficulty with dressing tasks due to apraxia following a CVA?
    a. Set out clothing for the client in an area of the room without clutter
    b. Place all clothing items grouped together in one area (i.e. shirts in drawer, all pants hanging)
    c. Place a colored label on the top and inside of the back of the garment to help cue the client to garment orientation
    d. Leave written instructions on how to dress with pictures

161. Where should you record a change in the occupational therapy treatment plan?
    a. It should be part of a re-evaluation
    b. It should be noted in the progress note
    c. It should be written as a separate entry in the medical record
    d. It should be written as an addendum to the original treatment plan

162. What non-profit organization is concerned with the advancement of education and research in occupational therapy?
    a. AOTF
    b. AOTA
    c. NBCOT
    d. AOTCB

163. Which of the following is true regarding occupational therapy services covered under Medicare Part B?
    a. A three-day hospital stay is required prior to receiving services
    b. Coverage is for inpatient rehabilitation only
    c. Clients may receive services without a physician prescription
    d. There are cap spending limits on occupational therapy services

164. Frames of reference most commonly used in mental health settings include all of the following except:
    a. psychodynamic.
    b. cognitive disabilities.
    c. biomechanical.
    d. the Model of Human Occupation.

165. Which of the following is a common area of concern for clients with eating disorders?
    a. Poor time management
    b. Problem-solving issues
    c. Stress management issues
    d. Negative body Image

166. What activity would be best to use when working with a client who has dysmetria?
    a. Copying clapping patterns
    b. Folding napkins
    c. Wiping down tables in the dining room
    d. Collecting salt and pepper shakers from the dining room

167. What is the name of the government program that provides health coverage for low-income families who meet its qualifications?
  a. Point of Service Plan
  b. Medicare part A
  c. Medicare part B
  d. Medicaid

168. What is the type of insurance that provides managed care through contracts with healthcare providers who treat clients within the guidelines and restrictions of the plan?
  a. Health Management Organization
  b. Health Maintenance Organization
  c. Health Mediated Organization
  d. None of the above

169. Which of the following play activities would be best for a five-year-old girl with spina bifida?
  a. Dolls and puppets
  b. Pop beads
  c. Board games, such as Monopoly and Parcheesi
  d. Hangman

170. What type of actions will a client perform who is level 4 on the Allen Cognitive Level Screen?
  a. Postural actions
  b. Automatic actions
  c. Goal-directed actions
  d. Manual actions

171. On the first day at a job in an outpatient clinic, a COTA is asked to complete the billing for the previous week for a COTA who is no longer employed by the facility. The facility manager has provided the progress notes from the previous sessions and has asked the COTA to use her best judgment in figuring out what should be billed. How should the COTA proceed?
  a. Review the progress notes and figure out the billable units as best she can
  b. Explain to the supervisor that she cannot submit billing for treatment she has not provided, as it is not ethical
  c. Call the previous COTA and ask what the units should be and then complete the billing
  d. Do the billing as best she can using progress notes and reviewing past billing

172. In providing a home program for a 60-year-old client with amyotrophic lateral sclerosis, which of the following would be most important?
  a. A heavy regimen of strengthening exercises to maintain strength
  b. Energy conservation and assistive device training
  c. Joint protection
  d. Coordination exercises

173. Which best describes breaking an activity into steps and teaching it one step at a time?
  a. Activity analysis
  b. Problem solving
  c. Sensitization
  d. Chaining

174. How often does NBCOT certification need to be renewed?
    a. Every year
    b. Every two years
    c. Every three years
    d. Every four years

175. What is the name of the codes used by practitioners to describe treatment services when billing?
    a. ICD-9 codes
    b. CPT Codes
    c. DRG codes
    d. BTC codes

176. Which of the following is true regarding skilled occupational therapy treatment?
    a. It can be provided by anyone who has been trained by an occupational therapist
    b. It is provided by nursing as part of a restorative occupational therapy program
    c. It can be provided by an occupational therapist, occupational therapy assistant, or an occupational therapy aide
    d. It can only be provided by an occupational therapist or by an occupational therapy assistant who is under the supervision of an occupational therapist

177. When working with a client in cardiac rehabilitation who is status post-myocardial infarction, activity should be slowed or stopped when resting heart rate is over:
    a. 120 bpm.
    b. 115 bpm.
    c. 110 bpm.
    d. 100 bpm.

178. What is the name of the unwritten rules in a group that govern how an individual behaves?
    a. Group processes
    b. Group rules
    c. Group norms
    d. Group dynamics

179. The monitoring and review of the care that is provided to clients with the goal of improving effectiveness of services is known as:
    a. utilization review.
    b. quality improvement.
    c. health care review.
    d. chart review.

180. When must documentation completed by a COTA be cosigned by an OTR?
    a. When it is required by an employer
    b. When it is required by the payer source
    c. When it is required by the regulatory board where the COTA is practicing
    d. All of the above

181. What type of instruction would be most effective to introduce cutting with scissors to a child with dyspraxia?
    a. Demonstration only
    b. Visual cueing
    c. Hand over hand with verbal cueing
    d. Verbal instruction

182. The evaluation and breakdown of components of an activity in order to choose and grade the activity for a client is called:
    a. performance components.
    b. activity analysis.
    c. therapeutic technique.
    d. occupational performance.

183. While working on transfers with a client, the client falls. What is the first thing that should be done?
    a. Fill out an incident report
    b. Ensure the safety of the client and do not move the client until he is checked for injuries
    c. Try to get the client into a chair and then go to get help
    d. Call a code or 911, depending on the setting

184. What should you do if you make an error in documentation?
    a. Tear out the page of the medical record and start over
    b. Use correction fluid and correct the error
    c. Cross over the error so it is not visible and continue writing
    d. Strike out the error, note the error, and initial it

185. Which of the following is an example of a re-entry program?
    a. Back to school
    b. Caregiver training
    c. Community education
    d. Vocational readiness

186. Initial certification for occupational therapy services provided by Medicare must be signed by a client's physician:
    a. within 30 days of initial treatment.
    b. before the initial evaluation is completed.
    c. after the initial evaluation, but before treatment can be initiated.
    d. at the end of the fiscal period.

187. Which of the following is true regarding early intervention services?
    a. Services are based on family-centered care
    b. Services are provided for children aged 0 to 6 years
    c. The written plan for services in early intervention is called an IEP
    d. Children identified can be treated without parental consent

188. What is the name of the Act signed into law in 2010 which was created to improve existing healthcare quality and to provide coverage to the uninsured?
   a. HIPAA
   b. HCFA
   c. ADA
   d. ACA

189. Why is clinical documentation necessary?
   a. It provides a legal record if needed
   b. It provides a clinical record of services
   c. It provides a record for financial reimbursement for services
   d. All of the above

190. What are the values, beliefs, and customs of a client known as?
   a. Culture
   b. Social beliefs
   c. Intrinsic factors
   d. Psychological factors

191. While working with a client with schizophrenia who is level 4 on ACLS, you ask him to make a ham and cheese sandwich. The client attempts to make the sandwich, but becomes frustrated early on. What should you do to modify the treatment session?
   a. Stop the activity and try something else
   b. Provide verbal cues while the client makes the sandwich
   c. End the treatment session
   d. Demonstrate how to make the sandwich and give the client the one you have made as a sample to copy

192. A client is receiving occupational therapy for chronic low back pain. She has been educated on proper body mechanics and lifting techniques as well as modifications at home. She reports that she will be returning part-time to her position as an administrative assistant in two weeks. What modifications would you recommend?
   a. She may want to explore other career opportunities
   b. Keep the keyboard at a level with elbows flexed to 45 degrees and wrists in neutral position or lightly extended
   c. Use a lumbar support and change positions every 20 minutes
   d. Stand up every 5-10 minutes and refuse to lift anything over 5 pounds

193. A progressive interdisciplinary rehabilitation program designed to help a client return to work through addressing various aspects of an occupation, including psychological, physical, functional, and vocational components is called a(n):
   a. ergonomic program.
   b. functional capacity program.
   c. occupational preparation program.
   d. work hardening program.

194. The technique of using empathy is best shown in which of the following responses to a pediatric client who is upset over a broken toy?
    a. "It's not that big of a deal."
    b. "I bet that makes you really sad that the toy is broken."
    c. "You really didn't play with that toy anyway."
    d. "It's all right; you have plenty of other toys to play with."

195. In an acute care setting, when should discharge planning be initiated?
    a. Immediately
    b. After initial evaluation
    c. When the physician indicates that the client will be discharged
    d. After the first few treatment sessions

196. Entry-level occupational therapy practitioners are those with:
    a. Less than one year of experience.
    b. Less than two years of experience
    c. Less than three years of experience.
    d. Less than five years of experience.

197. What is the main symptom noted in Asperger's syndrome?
    a. Decreased cognitive skills
    b. Decreased or absent language development
    c. Hyperactivity
    d. Poor social skills

198. Which of the following disorders is classified as an anxiety disorder?
    a. Post-traumatic stress disorder
    b. Dissociative identity disorder
    c. Borderline personality disorder
    d. Conduct disorder

199. Where are the receptors for the vestibular system located?
    a. In the cerebellum
    b. In the inner Ear
    c. In the medulla oblongata
    d. In the eye

200. Which of the following statements is true regarding parallel play?
    a. It involves an organized group with a goal
    b. Children involved participate in independent activities
    c. One child is watching others play
    d. Children play alongside each other but not with one another

Answers and Explanations

1. B: The biomechanical frame of reference is based on the belief that purposeful activities can be used to treat decreased range of motion, strength, and endurance.

2. A: The rehabilitative frame of reference teaches clients ways to become independent when deficits will not improve. Teaching a client to use compensatory strategies and adaptive equipment is would be utilizing the rehabilitation frame of reference.

3. D: A COTA may collect necessary data for a screening. A screening is a collection of data about a client to determine if there is a need for a comprehensive occupational therapy evaluation. A screening may include a record review, client/caregiver interview, and client observation. Screening data collection may be performed by a COTA after the OTR has established COTA competency for such tasks. Once data is collected, it is the responsibility of the OTR to analyze the data and to determine if an evaluation is indicated.

4. C: Once a COTA has established service competency, the OTR may assign the task of administering and scoring a standardized test. The COTA may also collect data through record reviews, checklists and interviews. A COTA cannot interpret test results or the need for intervention based on standardized test results.

5. C: The axis of the goniometer is placed on the axis of movement. The axis for elbow flexion is the lateral epicondyle of the humerus.

6. B: Desensitization programs should be graded from soft to hard materials. Light touch should be introduced first, followed by rubbing, tapping, and finally contact for an extended period of time. Cotton balls may be used to initiate the program and the stimulus should increase in pressure in accordance to client tolerance. Desensitization should be guided by the therapist but carried out by the client.

7. A: The soap dish is not secure enough to sustain the weight of a person transferring. The client must be educated that this is an unsafe practice that can lead to a fall or a serious injury. In order to perform safe transfers into a tub or shower, the client requires properly-installed grab bars and education on how to perform transfers safely in and out of the shower while using the grab bar.

8. B: If a client continues an activity to the point of fatigue, it may be very difficult to regain energy to complete a task. Principles of energy conservation include educating clients to rest before they become tired.

9. A: A client with a spinal cord injury needs to develop a tolerance for sitting. If raised to a sitting position too quickly, the client may faint, as his blood is not pumping efficiently and can pool in the lower extremities. This is called orthostatic hypotension. Tilting the wheelchair back so that the feet are higher than the head will help return the blood flow. This position should be maintained until the symptoms are no longer present. Orthostatic hypotension can be the result of changing positions too quickly or moving from supine to sitting.

10. C: The development of grasp begins with grasp independent of other motions (such as reach). The child's arm needs to be stabilized with the wrist in a neutral position in order to isolate grasping. The object needs to be placed in the child's hand, as reaching would require additional skills and is to be incorporated after grasp is present.

11. B: Following a total hip replacement, a patient cannot flex the hip of the operated leg past 90 degrees, cross his legs, or internally rotate the affected leg. Failure to follow total hip precautions can result in dislocation of the joint. Bending over from a seated position can cause flexion of the hip to exceed 90 degrees. Crossing the legs to put on socks is also contraindicated. Training in the use of adaptive equipment allows the patient to perform dressing tasks while observing total hip precautions.

12. D: Rheumatoid arthritis (RA) is a chronic inflammatory disease of the synovium of the joints characterized by exacerbations and remissions. Treatment during exacerbations should consist of preventing deformity through splinting and positioning, active and passive range of motion, energy conservation, joint protection education, adaptive equipment education, and stress management. The use of strengthening exercises such as progressively resistant exercises and isometrics should be avoided during inflammatory periods of RA.

13. C: Direct services are provided when an occupational therapy practitioner works with a student or a small group of students. Direct services are provided when the students' needs require the expertise of an occupational therapy practitioner for effective intervention.

14. D: A resting hand splint is used following a burn to prevent deformity in the hand. This splint is usually constructed in the intrinsic plus position, which is the wrist in extension, MP joints in flexion, and PIP and DIP joints in extension.

15. C: Splints need to be monitored for pressure areas, edema, and a client's physical changes that may require adjustments. Education of the client and caregiver on the splinting schedule, how to perform skin checks after wearing, and to report any issues with the splint is essential.

16. C: The Health Insurance Portability and Accountability Act of 1996 (HIPAA) protects an individual's identifiable health information. Sharing information on a crowded elevator allows all people present to have access to confidential information. Information that identifies an individual and his medical information should never be discussed in a public area or around other people.

17. A: Weighted utensils provide added input to the muscles and can help decrease extra movements associated with tremors and dyskinesia. This allows the client to improve accuracy for movements and decrease spills during self-feeding tasks.

18. B: Apraxia is being unable to carry out or execute movements even though a person wants to perform the movement. Apraxia is not due to a motor or sensory impairment, but it is a result of the inability to plan a motor activity. There are many different forms of apraxia. Ideational, ideomotor, and constructional apraxia are three types of apraxia that can interfere with activities of daily living.

19. D: The neurodevelopmental approach uses weight-bearing techniques to help decrease tone in an upper extremity with spasticity. In utilizing weight-bearing techniques, one must be sure that the extremity is in a proper position to prevent injury and to facilitate proper weight bearing. This is accomplished through positioning the shoulder in abduction (several inches away from the hip)

and external rotation. The elbow, wrist, and digits should be in extension. It is important to make sure that the client is not experiencing any pain or edema when weight bearing.

20. A: A client with a lesion at C6 can utilize a universal cuff for feeding and grooming activities. An injury at this level will not have hand and wrist motions, but may have radial wrist extension. The muscles for some shoulder, elbow, and forearm movements are being innervated, allowing for function with the assistance of adaptive devices for grasp.

21. D: Both the mobile arm support/balanced forearm orthoses and a suspension sling can help a client with significant upper extremity weakness. The mobile arm support/balanced forearm orthoses use gravity along with the shoulder and elbow muscles to perform motions of the elbow and forearm. This device has several adjustments to meet each client's needs. A suspension sling is also used to assist with shoulder and elbow motions. A suspension sling can also be adjusted in order to assist each client's needs.

22. B: The Americans with Disabilities Act (ADA) of 1990 is a civil rights law that ensures people with disabilities are given equal opportunities in regards to employment, public accommodations, transportation, government services, and telecommunications.

23. A: Phantom pain is a condition where the client who has suffered an amputation still feels as if the limb is there and experiences pain in that limb. This pain interferes with a client's ability to use a prosthetic. Treatment of phantom pain often requires intervention from multiple members of the treatment team.

24. B: Supervision means that the client needs someone with them to ensure they are performing an activity safely and correctly. Clients with decreased balance, decreased cognition, or diminished safety awareness are often at a supervision level. If a client requires physical assistance to perform the activity, then they are rated at a level of minimal assistance or lower.

25. A: When initiating transfer training with a client who has hemiparesis, it is easier to transfer with the stronger side leading. A pivot transfer is a good method of training as long as the client is able to bear weight on one or both lower extremities. After the client is able to transfer with the non-involved side leading, he should have training with the involved side leading, as there will be situations where the client is in a position where he must transfer that way.

26. C: A client who has intact triceps and can perform scapular depression should be trained to perform an independent depression transfer. This transfer would allow for the maximum level of independence.

27. A: Initially, energy conservation and work simplification tasks will need to be incorporated in order for the client to increase independence and work within her medical limitations. Quality of life can be improved by incorporating breathing techniques as well as energy conservation and work simplification techniques.

28. B: Since the client would be returning home alone, it is not safe for her to return at her current level of function. She still has a potential to improve, so long-term care would not be appropriate. She would not be safe at home alone even with home therapy or home health aides. An inpatient sub-acute unit at a rehabilitation facility would be the best option, as it could continue to work on her goals while providing 24-hour supervision.

29. D: Unilateral neglect is the failure to recognize or attend to the affected side. Often seen in right brain lesions, clients with neglect are often unaware of the affected side of the body as well as the space on the affected side. Homonymous hemianopsia is a visual field deficit that cuts the field of vision. The client can compensate for this vision loss by turning his head. Apraxia is difficulty with motor planning. Visual agnosia is the inability to recognize objects although vision is intact.

30. B: Standing with one foot on a stool will relieve pressure on the low back. Bending the knees when leaning over the sink is also taking pressure away from the back. Any bending done will put unwanted strain on the back. It is not realistic or comfortable to complete the entire task with the knees bent while at the sink. Performing this task while seated does not necessarily improve back mechanics.

31. A: Spreading the feet apart increases the base of support, which can help a person maintain balance. When working with a client who has decreased balance, educating him to widen his stance during standing activities can help to maintain balance.

32. B: Carpal tunnel syndrome is caused by compression of the median nerve at the carpal ligament. Symptoms include sensory impairment of digits 1, 2, and 3, and half of digit 4. Pain and weakness are also noted. Phalen's test is used as an indicator of median nerve compression at the carpal ligament. This test is positive when holding the wrist in a flexed position for one minute causes tingling or paresthesia.

33. C: Boutonniere deformity is caused by the stretch or tear of the central slip. This deformity is characterized by the DIP joint in hyperextension and the PIP joint in flexion.

34. D: A gel cushion is indicated due to the history of skin breakdown and the client's inability to perform weight shifting independently. Due to the diagnosis of MS, it is possible that the client's sensation is impaired and she cannot feel when she needs to perform weight shifting. Another type of cushion that would be suitable is an air cushion (i.e. ROHO). Foam cushions do very little to relieve pressure.

35. B: Reflex sympathetic dystrophy (RSD) is characterized by pain, edema, color changes in the skin, and temperature changes. The pain of RSD is often disproportionate to the injury and clients with this diagnosis are often hesitant to try to move. The use of passive stretch is contraindicated, as it will increase pain and discourage movement. Initial focus for a client with RSD is to decrease pain and edema. Active range of motion and gentle PROM should be used to increase range of motion.

36. C: Handwriting difficulties can be due to many factors. Improper position of the wrist and hand can make handwriting tasks difficult as well as increase the amount of work required to complete the tasks. The wrist should be in extension for writing and the use of a slanted writing surface can promote proper positioning for handwriting tasks. A dynamic quadruped grip is an efficient grip for writing, so a pencil grip is not needed. Using increased pressure for handwriting tasks can cause muscles to fatigue quickly. The use of a mechanical pencil can provide feedback for a client who uses too much pressure to write (lead will break with too much pressure) and can help the client adapt to use less pressure.

37. A: Noise-blocking headphones can help a student maintain focus as well as prevent a negative reaction to auditory input. Removing a student from the room or changing classrooms is not a realistic solution, as noise is often difficult to control and cannot always be predicted. Headphones

will still allow the student to hear, but can filter out additional sounds. These can be worn at certain times of the day or as needed. Other techniques to aid this student would be to give advanced notice before certain sounds (i.e. school bell, fire bell, announcements).

38. D: Slow rocking is inhibiting. Slow, rhythmical movements have been shown to decrease tone. Tapping, vibration, and icing are all techniques to facilitate muscle tone.

39. B: Brushing the lips is a facilatory technique that will increase lip closure.

40. C: A COTA is allowed to administer standardized tests as long as competency has been established. If standardized testing procedures are not followed for administration of the test, it can change the validity and reliability of the test scores.

41. B: Any stimulus that causes a negative response, such as the withdrawal response to pain, should not be used in attempts to increase a brain-injured client's response. Stimulation should be structured and various types can be used. Tactile, gustatory, visual, auditory, olfactory, and vestibular inputs can all be used to increase response.

42. D: Input that the brain receives from muscles and joints is interpreted to tell us where our bodies are in space. This sense is called proprioception. The tactile system makes us aware of touch. The visual system is responsible for what we see and the vestibular system is responsible for balance and the speed of movement.

43. A: When measuring wrist extension, the axis of the goniometer is placed on the radial styloid. The stationary arm is placed parallel to the radius and the moving arm is placed parallel to the longitudinal axis of the second metacarpal.

44. D: The vestibular system is responsible for our sense of motion and balance. The motion of swinging provides vestibular input. Some other examples of vestibular input are rocking, running, rolling, and jumping on a trampoline.

45. B: The asymmetrical tonic neck reflex is present from birth to 4 months. Often following a neurological injury, such as CVA or TBI, the reflex can be elicited. The asymmetrical tonic neck reflex is evidenced by flexion of the upper extremities and extension of the lower extremities when the neck is flexed.

46. C: Reflex sympathetic dystrophy is a condition where the pain is disproportionate to the injury. Symptoms often seen include pain, edema, changes in the appearance of the skin, and joint stiffness from disuse. Clients with RSD have an increased pain response to sensory input and can benefit from desensitization programs.

47. C: Working on an activity in the prone position helps improve extensors of the trunk. A child with flaccid cerebral palsy has decreased postural strength. The use of standing frames and being seated at a table provides assistance to the postural muscles, but are not as challenging.

48. B: Tenderness in the calf when touched, edema, and pain upon passive dorsiflexion are all symptoms of deep venous thrombosis (DVT). Clients who are post-CVA are at risk for DVT as they are often in bed and have decreased activity. Reporting findings to the nurse or physician for follow-up testing is imperative. Patients with DVT are at risk for pulmonary embolism, which can be fatal.

49. C: The quadruped position provides the most input while weight bearing on a spastic upper extremity. Weight shifting in this position increases the amount of input. Completing activities while standing and seated are used to incorporate weight bearing as well.

50. A: The use of reach requires moving the center of gravity and therefore increases the challenge to maintain balance. Adding weights increases the resistance to muscles. Weights can sometimes be incorporated to challenge balance but it is dependent on the activity.

51. A: Decreased internal rotation of the shoulders makes putting on and taking off a bra very difficult. A front-closure bra is easier to put on and close. Compensatory strategies for dressing can also assist a person who has decreased range of motion to put on and take off both cardigan and overhead shirts.

52. C: A three-in-one commode is a versatile piece of durable medical equipment. It can be used bedside, over a standard commode, and in the shower. It is not indicated to be used as a chair for tub transfers.

53. C: While all the activities listed can be used to improve standing endurance, it is important to remember that activity selection should be meaningful to a client. XBOX games would be best used with a younger population. Coloring a picture could be insulting to an adult, as coloring is often associated with children. Nuts and bolts would most likely be better suited for a male client. It is always important to find out what types of activities hold meaning to a client and choose activities that would be interesting. If the client is actively engaged in the activity, it will increase the benefit.

54. A: In order to promote proper tone and to prevent contractures and subluxation, pillows should be placed under the affected shoulder and the affected hip.

55. C: A muscle that is graded Poor minus cannot move through full range on a gravity-eliminated plane. A person with this muscle grade would not be able to perform exercises against gravity (with or without resistance). The use of an arm skate on a table eliminates gravity and allows the muscle to perform work to improve strength.

56. B: Systolic blood pressure will increase as a result of the body's increased demands for oxygen. Diastolic blood pressure is a measure of the pressure of the blood vessels between heartbeats and will therefore not change.

57. C: Armrest height is measured from the seat to the elbow (flexed 90 degrees), and then one inch is added. This promotes a proper height in which to rest the arms for proper posture.

58. B: Activities in cardiac rehabilitation work on strengthening the heart muscle while simultaneously allowing the heart to heal. Activities such as walking for 20 minutes on a treadmill improve stamina and circulation. Climbing stairs is an activity to slowly work into, but this should be done at home and not in a large, steep area. Hot and cold temperatures increase the demands of an activity. Sitting in a hot and humid environment such as a sauna or doing excessive work in cold temperatures, such as shoveling snow, may be contraindicated for months following a myocardial infarction.

59. A: A client who is having difficulty with moving his body in space and is bumping into others is often having difficulty with body awareness. An obstacle course would allow this client to practice

- 95 -

movement control around the obstacles. This allows for practice of several types of movements while learning to adapt movements for different situations quickly. Obstacles will assist with feedback to the client as to proper positioning and activity demands.

60. A: Visual reminders can help orient a client to time and place. When a client is first admitted to a new care facility, it is important to establish routine and to help with the adjustment. As a routine is set, a client may have a better understanding of what to expect. Caregivers should always approach a client in a calm manner, explaining to the client why they are there.

61. B: A weighted lap pad provides proprioceptive input to help maintain a seated position. A weighted blanket also provides this input but is not appropriate for use at a desk. Fidget toys and chewy toys provide tactile and oral motor input, which would not be as effective in helping a student stay in her seat.

62. D: Sensory avoiding is a term that was developed by Winnie Dunn and describes clients who are hypersensitive to a particular type of sensory input. These clients are often very aware of input and may limit behaviors that cause increased sensory input. This can manifest as being defensive and uncooperative when expected to participate in group activities.

63. D: Total hip precautions state that a client cannot flex the hip of the operated leg past 90 degrees, cross the legs, or internally rotate the affected leg. The amount of time a client must adhere to precautions is determined by the surgeon. The usual amount of time is around six weeks, but can vary based on the surgeon and the client's status.

64. B: The left side of the brain is responsible for language. Injury to the left side can affect both speech and language. The right side of the brain is responsible for memory and perception.

65. B: Ice massage can be used in the acute phase of lateral epicondylitis to decrease pain. Heat may increase swelling and resistive exercise can increase inflammation and stress to the tendon.

66. C: It is important to block the knees of a client when performing a stand pivot transfer. If the client's knees buckle during a transfer; it will increase the workload and can put both the client and the person assisting with the transfer at risk for injury.

67. C: When performing transfers, a therapist must always assess the situation. If for any reason a therapist feels that he may not be able to assist the client independently, he should always seek help. If in the middle of a transfer, a therapist is unable to complete the transfer, it can result in injury to both the client and the therapist.

68. C: Universal precautions must be followed when coming into contact with body fluids.

69. D: Brunnstrom's flexor synergy of the upper extremity consists of shoulder retraction and elevation, shoulder abduction and external rotation, supination of the forearm, and elbow flexion.

70. D: A splint worn at night will not interfere with functional use and can prevent risk of contractures in the position the hand is in throughout the night.

71. A: The D1 flexion pattern is used when brushing hair to the opposite side as the shoulder is in adduction, flexion, and external rotation. The elbow is flexed and the digits are flexed and adducted.

72. C: The wrapping method of a residual limb is extremely important as it helps shape the limb to be able to tolerate a prosthetic in the future. Using the figure-eight pattern helps to mold the stump and maintain even pressure for edema control. The limb should be wrapped from the proximal to the distal end in the figure-eight pattern.

73. C: ADL training should be done both with and without a prosthesis in a client with an above-the-knee amputation. There will be times when an amputee may not be able to wear the prosthetic, so it is necessary to ensure independence for situations when this may occur.

74. A: Providing carpet squares will provide each child with physical boundaries and prevent unintentional touch. Removing the student is restrictive and does not allow him to participate in his educational program. A reward system would not be effective, as tactile defensive reactions are not a behavior. Asking children to sit away from the client would not be that effective, as students would have difficulty maintaining space. This would also isolate the student in the classroom, which should be avoided.

75. A: Instrumental activities of daily living are those that are more complex than ADLs. ADLs are basic activities of self-care, mobility, and communication. IADLs include home management and community living. Meal preparation is considered an IADL. Shaving, opening a door, and brushing the teeth are all considered ADLs.

76. D: Constructional apraxia is the inability to copy or construct a design. This is often seen in clients with histories of CVA or head injuries. Ideational apraxia is the inability to perform a motor task automatically or when asked to do something. Ideomotor apraxia is the inability to perform a task that is not automatic. Dressing apraxia is seen when a client is unable to perform dressing tasks or performs them incorrectly.

77. B: When working with a client who has ideational apraxia, it is best to work on each step individually with repetition before trying to perform the entire task. Tactile and verbal instructions can be helpful when working with a client with ideational apraxia. Lengthy verbal instructions and demonstrations are not effective.

78. C: Applied behavior analysis uses the behavioral approach to shape wanted behaviors and fade unwanted behaviors. Reinforcement is used in this treatment approach.

79. D: An isometric contraction does not involve movement of the joint and the muscle length is unchanged. Isotonic contractions, also known as concentric contractions, involve movement of a joint and the muscle shortens. An eccentric contraction involves joint motion with lengthening of the muscle.

80. B: Open wounds should not be placed in paraffin as it increases the risk for infection to the client and may contaminate the paraffin.

81. C: When performing passive range of motion for a person with quadriplegia it is important to extend the wrist while flexing the fingers and to flex the wrist while extending the fingers, so that the tendons are never fully stretched.

82. D: A doorway must be at least 32 inches wide to allow a wheelchair to pass through it.

83. C: The stage 3 motor response on the Glasgow Coma Scale is known as abnormal flexion or decorticate rigidity. In a decorticate response, the trunk extends; the knees and hips are stiff and extended. The arms are bent at the elbow with the wrists and fingers flexed on the chest.

84. D: As a part of joint protection, you should always stop a painful activity to avoid further aggravation to the joint. Holding a joint in a sustained position is to be avoided as well. Planning ahead and taking rest breaks are principles of work simplification.

85. A: Using larger and stronger joints is a principle of joint protection.

86. B: Multiple sclerosis symptoms can be exacerbated by changes in temperature, including very hot or very cold temperature fluctuations. These temperature changes are known as triggers, which may cause a flare of MS symptoms such as blurred vision or muscle spasticity.

87. B: Rheumatoid arthritis is a systemic disease characterized by pain, swelling, decreased movement, and inflammation. The inflammation is in the joints and there are periods of flare-ups and remissions. Joint deformities are often the result of flare-ups. One deformity seen with rheumatoid arthritis of the hands is ulnar drift of the MP joints due to laxity of the ligaments. Splinting and joint protection can help prevent these deformities.

88. B: Modulation is how information that is received is regulated by the nervous system to form a response. Modulation allows a person to respond appropriately to necessary information while disregarding irrelevant information. Modulation can affect alertness and the ability to maintain attention to a task. Difficulties with modulation can be classified as over-responsive, under-responsive, and sensory-seeking.

89. B: Lateral supports provide support for the lateral trunk. These supports are used to prevent the client from leaning to either side. An abduction wedge is often used to maintain lower extremity position and to prevent a client from sliding forward out of a chair. A firm seat insert can prevent the seat from slinging in the middle which affects seated position. Detachable arm rests are often helpful for performing certain types of transfers.

90. C: The S in a soap note is for the subjective report of the patient. Other parts of the note include the objective information (O), assessment (A), and the plan (P).

91. A: A splint-wearing schedule should always be given to the client as part of a home splinting program. A client should not be instructed on modifications but rather should be educated to contact the therapist if there are any difficulties with the splint. The material and the pattern used to make the splint is information that the client does not need.

92. C: The clock method would be best for assisting a client when there is a caregiver available. When utilizing the clock method, descriptions of food at clock positions are given. For example: chicken at 12 o'clock, peas at 3 o'clock, and rice at 6 o'clock.

93. B: A client who is at level V on the Ranchos Los Amigos Scale has a confused, inappropriate response. This client is alert but will not initiate activities. At this level, a client requires structure and direction to perform activities. The client at this stage can follow simple commands but cannot respond appropriately to complex directions or those without structure. At this stage, agitation can still be present and there is a high level of distractibility. Supervision is required for feeding tasks.

94. A: A client who is at level III of the Rancho Los Amigos Scale is able to perform simple one-step activities, which require making a choice between two objects (i.e. pick the red circle when given a choice between two colors). The goal at this level is to improve consistency and speed of responses. Ten-piece puzzles, crosswords, and complex block designs would be too difficult at this stage.

95. B: Licensure to practice occupational therapy is governed by individual states. In order to practice in a state, an application must be made with that state's licensing agency. Passing the certification test does not allow a therapist or assistant to practice as a licensed therapist.

96. B: Low lighting in a room can affect a client's ability to navigate through an area and to see potential hazards that can result in falls. Poor posture and ear infections can also contribute to falls, but these are not environmental factors.

97. A: The optimal position for feeding is upright with the hips at a 90-degree angle. This can be achieved by raising the head of the bed. This position ensures safe swallowing and prevents reflux. A client should maintain this position for at least 10-20 minutes after a meal.

98. D: A nosey cup allows a person with decreased flexion to drink while maintaining proper swallowing position. The cup is angled so that a person can tip the cup without obstruction from the nose. A weighted cup is indicated for a person who may have difficulties due to tremors or coordination issues. Using a taller cup would prove more difficult, as it is harder to tilt the cup. A T-shaped mug is used for decreased grasp.

99. C: An occupational therapy aide is able to perform specific client tasks once training and competency is completed. An aide can be supervised by an OTR or a COTA. An OT aide is not to perform skilled occupational therapy intervention, as he or she is not trained to make clinical judgments and cannot judge what is required to adapt certain activities.

100. B: A wedge cushion could help the client remain seated safely while being the least restrictive. A full lap tray and the use of a seatbelt are considered restraints and should not be used to promote a least restrictive environment. Anti-tippers stop the wheel chair from tipping over, which was not an issue for this client.

101. B: Email messaging and written communications are considered indirect supervision. Observation, co-treatment, and meetings are all considered direct supervision. The type of supervision that is required may vary by practice setting, the complexity of clients, and regulatory rules. Needs should be determined based on appropriate and safe delivery of OT services.

102. B: Clients with figure-ground difficulties often have issues with finding something that is in a group of items. Color-coding books can help distinguish one thing from another. Other techniques that can help include using organizational containers, removing clutter, and using an organizational checklist.

103. D: Ripping paper requires integration of both sides of the body to complete the activity. Decoupage would also be a good choice as an age-appropriate activity. Pinching Theraputty, painting, and card games do not require both sides of the body to work together and therefore would not be the best activities to work on bilateral integration.

104. B: If a client is no longer making progress and the COTA feels that the client will no longer make progress in a sub-acute setting, the COTA should collaborate with the OT regarding discharge. Together, the COTA and OTR can make appropriate discharge recommendations.

105. A: The Code of Ethics was established by the AOTA to be used as a guide to promote and maintain ethical behavior. The Code of Ethics applies to all occupational therapy personnel and students.

106. A: Emotional lability is the result of injury to the areas of the brain that regulate emotional activity, often following a CVA or traumatic brain injury. Clients with emotional lability often have emotions (crying, laughing, irritability) that are out of proportion to the situation.

107. C: A client with a spinal cord injury at C8/T1 is able to get around with a standard wheelchair. This client is able to utilize upper extremities for self-care as well as participate in sports at the wheelchair level. The client may participate in all activities listed, but basketball would be the best choice, as he was previously active and this would allow him to continue to participate in athletic activities.

108. B: A client with an injury at C6 may be able to use hand controls to operate a vehicle. Injuries above C6 are not able to use hand controls efficiently.

109. B: Self-assessment is used to help determine what type of stress management program is needed for an individual. Self-assessment is used to help identify what triggers stress in an individual. All other answer choices are methods of stress management.

110. C: The Americans with Disabilities Act (ADA) was passed in 1990, stating that businesses with more than 15 employees must be accessible to persons with disabilities.

111. A: Retrograde massage followed by active range of motion would be the best initial activities for this client. The active range of motion exercises are used instead of passive exercises, as they can help decrease edema through their pumping action as well as improve the client's range and strength. Functional activities are also beneficial, but controlling and increasing range of motion would be of more benefit to the client initially. Instruction in home programs to include retrograde massage, AROM, and other edema-control techniques are also necessary.

112. D: An environmental control unit (ECU) is used to help a person with physical limitations operate electronic devices such as lamps, televisions, and appliances. These units may be stand-alone or they may work through a computer software program. ECUs may be controlled by a switch or they may be voice-controlled.

113. A: The Representative Assembly is composed of representatives from each state and those abroad who are elected. The Representative Assembly makes the policy and legislative decisions. The Executive Board has a hired executive director and is responsible for management of the AOTA. There are three commissions that are under the direction of the Executive Board and the Representative Assembly. They are the Commission on Education, the Commission on Standards and Ethics, and the Commission on Practice.

114. D: Osteogenesis imperfecta is an orthopedic condition also known as brittle bones. Children who are diagnosed with this condition suffer from frequent fractures. Extra care must be taken to be gentle when working with a client diagnosed with osteogenesis imperfecta.

115. B: A typical child is able to sit unsupported by the age of 9 months. Independent sitting at this age does not require an increased base of support and weight shifting is used to reach for things.

116. A: Picking up Cheerios requires the use of tip pinch.

117. C: A curved spoon can be used to help get food to the mouth when wrist ROM is limited. The use of built-up handles will also assist a child with decreased finger ROM and decreased grasp.

118. B: Ergonomics is the science of equipment design and workplace factors to optimize productivity while decreasing the risk of injury and illness. Ergonomic programs are used to prevent injury and illness in the workplace through worksite analysis, hazard control, medical management, and worker training and education.

119. D: The force required for a job, positions used to complete a job (sustained and those that are awkward), and repetitive motions can all be causes of cumulative trauma injuries. Shift work is not a causative factor for cumulative trauma.

120. C: Cerebral palsy classified as athetosis presents with fluctuations in tone, writhing movements, and observed protective reactions. Spastic cerebral palsy usually presents with increased tone, slow movements, and primitive reflexes. Flaccid cerebral palsy presents with decreased tone, hypermobile joints, and delayed or decreased protective reactions. Ataxic cerebral palsy presents with normal (or near normal) tone and range of motion with uncoordinated movements and tremors at rest.

121. A: Self-inspection via the use of mirrors is vital in the prevention of decubitus ulcers, bruising, and fungal infections in a client with spinal cord injury. Clients with spinal cord injury are susceptible to skin breakdown due to decreased movement and decreased sensation. Increased pressure due to positioning as well as increased shearing forces will also increase the likelihood of skin breakdown and bruising. Maintaining hygiene is important to avoid fungal infections.

122. A: Cold does not necessarily increase the risk for decubitus ulcers. Heat, pressure, and shearing forces are all contributing factors to skin breakdown and decubitus ulcers.

123. C: Heterotopic ossification (HO) is the name given to the abnormal growth of bone following an injury or surgery. Some clients that may encounter HO include those with spinal cord injuries or burns, and those who have had hip replacement surgeries.

124. C: Copper tooling with a template is a good activity choice for clients in a mental health setting, as it ensures successful outcomes. Many clients in a mental health setting have decreased self-esteem and often fear failure. Copper tooling can be graded and is a simple craft that allows for choices. Copper tooling templates provide clear boundaries that can help a client maintain control.

125. A: When the wrist is in a neutral position, the least pressure is exerted on the median nerve at the carpal ligament.

126. D: Stereognosis is the ability to identify what an object is though tactile information. It is not describing the characteristics (such as soft or hard), but actually identifying what an object is. Stereognosis gives a person the ability to reach into a bag and pull out the item they want without having to look in the bag.

127. C: Following a total hip arthroplasty, modifications are required to observe hip precautions as well as account for deficits in strength and ROM following surgery. A person who has had a total hip replacement is able to transfer into a tub using grab bars and by bending the leg at the knee (vs. the hip) to get over the tub ledge. This type of transfer may be prove difficult and may increase the risk of falls for someone who has a history of falls. A tub transfer bench is the safer option that allows a person to transfer without the risk of falling, thereby maintaining hip precautions. A long-handled sponge and a shower hose will also allow for ease in bathing while observing precautions.

128. C: Twisting from side to side places increased stress on the spine ten times its normal amount of stress. Torsional stress, such as by twisting, places greater strain on the body than bending, reaching, or swaying.

129. A: Many clients with traumatic brain injuries suffer from decreased psychosocial skills as a result of their injuries. Interactions with peers in a group setting allow opportunities to work on social skills in a structured environment.

130. B: A prosthetic sock is worn under the prosthesis to protect the skin and to absorb perspiration. A client should wear a clean sock daily.

131. B: A volumeter is used to measure hand edema though the displacement of water. The hand is placed into the volumeter and water displaces into a beaker. The displaced water is then measured. Finger edema is usually measured through circumferential measures with a tape measure.

132. D: Retrieving the blue chips from a collection of various colored chips requires the client to visually discriminate blue from the other colors in the background using figure-ground perception.

133. C: Rehearsal is a strategy used to increase short-term memory by repeating the information over and over. Chunking is another method where information is grouped into smaller units for recall.

134. B: The wheelchair should be placed at a 45-degree angle for most transfers.

135. A: A client with COPD may have decreased strength endurance. Reaching and bending in the kitchen will require more work than getting things at the counter level. It is recommended that the items used most often be kept on the counter and others in the cabinets just above and just below. This technique of work simplification will make kitchen tasks much easier.

136. A: Deep pressure is calming to a child with tactile defensiveness.

137. D: While all of the suggestions may benefit a client with RA, the jar opener would be most beneficial. Opening jars requires hand strength that a client may not have during a rheumatoid arthritis exacerbation. It also requires force on the wrist joints, which is contraindicated for someone with this diagnosis. Using a jar opener can help protect the joints as well as simplify the task.

138. D: Taking apart pop beads is an age-appropriate activity that would provide a challenge but also allow for success. Stringing small beads is a good a bilateral upper extremity activity but it is not age-appropriate for skill level at 18 months. Finger-painting and copying block designs are good choices in order to work on bilateral integration.

139. A: Positive reinforcement provides a reward for wanted behaviors. In this case, the chips are an immediate reward and the prize the boys earn with the chips is the reward that provides motivation. An example of negative reinforcement would be to take chips away for unwanted behaviors. A time out would be an example of punishment.

140. A: When swallowing difficulties are suspected, the client may be at risk for developing aspiration pneumonia. It is appropriate to make a referral to a speech language pathologist to address any concerns with dysphagia.

141. C: Professional development units (PDUs) are a requirement to renew certification through the NBCOT every three years. State requirements regarding continuing education and professional development for license renewal vary among each jurisdiction.

142. B: State regulatory bodies regulate supervision requirements for occupational therapy assistants. Each state has different requirements, so both the OT and the OT assistant should be knowledgeable about the legislation regarding supervision in the state where they are practicing.

143. C: A single switch would be best as it would be easiest for him to operate with the least training requirements. The use of a joystick requires more controlled gross motor motions, but allows for more options. Keyboards can be used once pointing is achieved. With adapted techniques, improved skills, and additional time for training, other switch options are available for this client.

144. D: New staff orientation is not considered professional development by the NBCOT. Employer-sponsored professional development courses (including CPR) are considered professional development.

145. C: The NBCOT is a national certification that does not replace state requirements, but complements them. NBCOT regulations are the same for all practitioners, regardless of the state they practice in. The NBCOT provides initial credentials for OT practitioners through the certification exam and monitors continuing competence of practitioners through renewals. Each state jurisdiction has its own laws and regulations in regards to competency and license to practice.

146. C: Caregiver concerns must be considered in order to provide a continuum of care for a client. These concerns come up frequently and must be addressed by the treatment team. Social workers are vital in discharge planning and in most settings work with the therapist, client, and caregiver in finding the best placement after discharge.

147. B: Uniform Terminology for Occupational Therapy is an official document of the AOTA. Its purpose is to create common terminology among practitioners and to educate others about occupational therapy. There are three domains: performance areas, performance components, and performance concepts. Play is a performance area.

148. A: Cultural beliefs are a part of performance contexts (environmental aspects).

149. A: Any time a COTA does not feel he or she has the competence to treat a particular diagnosis; it should be discussed with the supervising OTR. Ethical practice requires a practitioner to provide services that he or she is competent to treat.

150. C: Certified occupational therapy assistants provide supervision for occupational therapy aides. They do not provide supervision for other occupational therapy assistants or new graduate occupational therapists, as these are the responsibilities of a supervising occupational therapist.

151. A: Evidence based practice is an important component of occupational therapy treatment. Evidence-based practice takes into account research evidence, a therapist's knowledge, and clinical judgment in order to provide the most effective treatment.

152. B: A wheelchair is considered durable medical equipment and is covered by Medicare with a physician prescription and when the client meets criteria. Reachers, transfer tub benches, and elastic laces are not considered durable medical equipment covered by Medicare.

153. B: Under the Code of Ethics principle 8.2, a sexual relationship with a current client, even when consensual, is a violation of the Code of Ethics. This also holds true for research participants, employees, and students.

154. B: When working with a client who has delusions, it is important to show empathy to the client and not to challenge delusional thoughts or increase defensiveness of the client.

155. B: When working with a client who has dementia, establishing a routine is necessary. Change is often upsetting to a client with dementia and can increase the stress on the caregiver. Routine helps the client maintain abilities and decreases confusion.

156. A: Since the client is at a level of modified independence in ADLs, he does not require inpatient therapy services. Because he is high functioning, reimbursement for services at an inpatient level may be denied. This client does require supervision for home management, which his wife is able to provide, so a home health aide is not necessary. The appropriate recommendation would be to discharge the client to home with a referral for outpatient therapy.

157. C: A long-term goal is the expected outcome at the time of discharge. Long-term goals should be measurable and functional. Answer choices A, B, and D are examples of short-term goals, which should also be measurable. Short-term goals should address problem areas and work toward achieving long-term goals.

158. D: The client response to treatment should always be included in a progress note. Other information that should be included in a progress note is the treatment the client received and the plan for services. Prior level of function and the referral source are included on the initial evaluation. The problem list is a part of the plan of care.

159. C: The problem oriented medical record (POMR) is a comprehensive approach to charting based on a master client problem list. In this type of record, an interdisciplinary plan of treatment is created instead of each discipline creating its own. Notes in the POMR are written in SOAP format and address the problems.

160. C: Clients with dressing apraxia often have difficulty orienting clothing and may put clothes on upside down or inside out. Using a label on a garment can help orient the client to how the clothing should be used for dressing tasks. An example would be to place the label on the inside of a garment at the top. The client would then know that the label side is the inside and the label should be at the top. Labels may also be placed to distinguish left from right.

161. B: Any changes to therapy treatment should be documented in the occupational therapy progress note.

162. A: The American Occupational Therapy Foundation (AOTF) is a non-profit organization that operates with a goal of advancing research, education, and the leadership of occupational therapy. The AOTF provides scholarships, recognizes research contributions, and works with the AOTA on research priorities and practice parameters.

163. D: Medicare part B is an outpatient payer. There are limits in the amount of money Medicare part B will pay for medically necessary outpatient services each year. This is referred to as a cap limitation. The cap amounts are determined by Medicare and there is one amount for occupational therapy and one for physical therapy and speech therapy combined. In 2013, the limit was $1900 for occupational therapy and $1900 for physical and speech therapy.

164. C: The frames of reference that are commonly used in mental health settings include: the Model of Human Occupation, psychodynamic, cognitive, sensory integration, and developmental. The biomechanical frame of reference is used in clients with physical disabilities and with pediatric populations.

165. D: An impaired body image is often the result of delusional thoughts of those with eating disorders. Body image is a primary treatment concern with clients who have eating disorders. Some ways body image is addressed in occupational therapy treatment is through reality testing, addressing clothing and appearance in ADLs, and education on the proper way to care for one's body.

166. D: Dysmetria is the inability to control muscle length. As a result, a person who has dysmetria will overshoot when trying to pick up an object. Picking up salt and pepper shakers allows a person to practice controlled tasks.

167. D: Medicaid is an insurance program for low-income individuals and families who qualify. Medicaid is funded by federal and state governments and also provides coverage for certain individuals with disabilities.

168. B: Health Maintenance Organizations (HMOs) provide managed care for their recipients though contracts with healthcare providers. The HMO will cover the cost of the services (at a contracted rate) for providers in exchange for providing the healthcare practitioner with clients. HMO clients usually have a primary care physician who will give a referral to a specialist if HMO guidelines deem that it is necessary. Therapy services require a referral under HMO guidelines.

169. A: Dolls and puppets would be the best choice for play therapy with a five-year-old girl with spina bifida. These are age-appropriate toys that would allow her to engage in creative play alone or with others. Pop beads are not appropriate as they are more suited for a younger child. Games like Monopoly and Parcheesi are for children who are older, as they require increased attention and cognition. Hangman is not appropriate for a five-year-old child, as it requires spelling.

170. C: A client who is level 4 on the Allen Cognitive Level Screen will perform goal-directed actions. A client at this level can carry out routines that are already established and engage in simple activities. Learning new skills at this level is accomplished by imitation or following a demonstration.

171. B: Billing for services not performed is unethical. The COTA who provided the services is the only one who can bill for services rendered. That COTA is the only one who knows exactly what services were provided as well as how long each service was provided. If the newly-hired COTA were to complete the billing, it would not only be a violation of the Code of Ethics, but would also be considered fraudulent billing and could be subject to regulatory and legal repercussions.

172. B: Amyotrophic lateral sclerosis (ALS) is a rapidly-progressive degenerative disease. Although the course is rapid, it is also variable. In working with a client with ALS, anticipation of further decline is necessary. In providing a home program education, work simplification and the use of adaptive devices is very important, as it will allow the client to maintain independence and continue participation in daily activities despite declining motor function. Strengthening exercises will also be a part of home exercise to maintain strength but must be mild as not to promote fatigue.

173. D: Chaining is a behavioral method of learning where a task is broken down into small steps and taught to the learner one step at a time. Reverse chaining is teaching one step at a time backwards (starting at the last step).

174. C: NBCOT certification needs to be renewed every three years. In order to complete renewal, you must complete professional development units.

175. B: Current Procedural Terminology codes (CPT codes) are owned by the American Medical Association. CPT codes are used to report the medical services and procedures. The CPT codes provide a uniform language that is used by healthcare providers, administrators, and payers.

176. D: Skilled occupational therapy is that treatment which can only be performed effectively by a trained occupational therapist or occupational therapy assistant working under the general supervision of a skilled therapist.

177. A: If the heart rate of a client who is post-myocardial infarction goes over 120 beats per minute during an activity, it is an abnormal response and the activity must be slowed or stopped. Other signs involving heart rate that would require a change in activity levels are failure of heart rate to return to resting rate 10 minutes after activity, no change in heart rate with increased activity, and an increase greater than 20 beats per minute over the resting rate.

178. C: Group norms are the unwritten rules for behavior in groups. These norms evolve in a group and are often a result of how the group leader models behavior. The group leader is also involved in redirecting unwanted behavior, which also contributes to the development of group norms.

179. B: Quality Improvement (QI) is the review of client care and services with the goal of improving the effectiveness of care provided.

180. D: Documentation that is completed by a COTA must be co-signed by an OTR when it is required by the employer, the payer source, and/or the regulatory board where the COTA is practicing.

181. C: Dyspraxia often results in difficulties with fine motor movements and movement patterns. A client with this diagnosis would have difficulty imitating the act of cutting after demonstration as well as following verbal cueing. Hand-over-hand techniques accompanied by verbal cueing provide a multisensory approach to learning that is best suited for this population.

182. B: Activity analysis is used by an occupational therapist to examine all the components of an activity and to examine how the activity can be graded to meet the right challenge for a client. Some of the components that may be examined in activity analysis are motor, sensory, cognitive, perceptual, social, and cultural.

183. B: You must always first ensure the safety of the patient. If a patient falls, you do not want to move him until he has been assessed for injuries. Moving an injured client may cause further injury. When a client falls, you must fill out documentation according to the facility guidelines. This usually requires an incident report. You will also want to note this in the therapy record as a method of communication to other professionals working with the client.

184. D: Whenever you make an error in documentation, you should strike a single line through it, note the error, and sign it. Using correction fluid, erasers, or scribbling over an error is not allowed.

185. D: A vocational readiness program can help a client re-enter the community as a worker following an illness or injury. These types of programs help the client gain the skills necessary to function in the community. Back to school, caregiver education, and community education programs are all part of health and wellness.

186. A: Initial certifications for Medicare must be signed by a physician within 30 days of the initial treatment.

187. A: Early intervention services are provided as part C of IDEA for infants and toddlers with a focus on family-centered care. The written plan of care in early intervention is called an Individual Family Service Plan (IFSP). Parental consent is required for early intervention services.

188. D: The Affordable Care Act was signed in March 2010 by President Obama. This Act was designed to improve existing healthcare and to provide health insurance to uninsured Americans.

189. D: Clinical documentation provides a clinical record of the services rendered. It also provides a record for legal and reimbursement purposes. Clinical documentation is a source of communication for providers to convey important information and to provide a continuum of care.

190. A: Values, beliefs, and customs are a part of a person's culture. Culture plays a vital role in the performance and needs of a client. It is important to incorporate culture into goals and treatment.

191. D: A client who is a level 4 on the ACLS does best with visual cues. Verbal cues alone would most likely not provide enough assistance for this client. When a client becomes frustrated with an activity, the therapist should decide if the activity can create the right challenge or if it should be discontinued. By providing a demonstration and visual cues, the client can experience success in the activity.

192. C: A client who is returning to work with chronic low back pain is best advised to use a lumbar support in order to provide support to the curves of the spine and to decrease pressure. If the client's job requires long periods of sitting, she should also be educated to take breaks about every twenty minutes to relieve the pressure from the prolonged position and to allow her to stretch.

193. D: Work hardening provides an individualized interdisciplinary approach to help a client return to work after illness or injury. Work hardening covers many aspects of job requirements and

uses graded simulated work activities that are progressive in order for the worker to return to the workforce.

194. B: Empathy is an important tool in therapeutic use of self. Empathy is being able to recognize what the client is feeling from his point of view. Recognizing what the client is feeling and making him aware that you are empathic to his feelings helps foster a more positive relationship.

195. A: In order to address all the needs of the client and to ensure appropriate discharge, discharge planning must be instituted as soon as the client is referred to services.

196. A: An entry-level practitioner (OTR or COTA) is one with less than one year of experience. There are guidelines regarding the practice and supervision of entry-level practitioners.

197. D: Asperger's syndrome is a disorder that is a part of the autism spectrum. Clients diagnosed with Asperger's typically have normal or near-normal cognitive and language development. One of the hallmark symptoms of Asperger's is difficulty with social interactions and non-verbal communication. Other symptoms that may be seen with Asperger's include repetitive behaviors, unusual interests, and difficulties with motor skills (awkward or clumsy).

198. A: Post-traumatic stress disorder (PTSD) is an anxiety disorder that develops after someone has witnessed or experienced something traumatic. Symptoms of PTSD can include anxiety, emotional arousal, avoidance, and reliving the traumatic event.

199. B: The receptors for the vestibular system are located in the inner ear. The vestibular system is the sensory system that is responsible for providing information about movement and balance.

200. D: Parallel play involves children playing next to each other, but not interacting with one another. In associative and cooperative play, children interact with one another. Other types of play include unoccupied, onlooker, and solitary play.